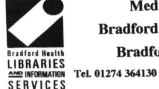

For JT and Madge Caulfield
and for Peter Wilkinson

The Human Rights Act

A Practical Guide for Nurses

ROSIE WILKINSON

Advisor in Nursing Practice – Acute Care and Ethics
at the Royal College of Nursing, London

AND

HELEN CAULFIELD

Solicitor and Health Policy Analyst
at the Royal College of Nursing, London

W

WHURR PUBLISHERS
LONDON AND PHILADELPHIA

© 2000 Whurr Publishers
First published 2000 by
Whurr Publishers Ltd
19b Compton Terrace, London N1 2UN, England and
325 Chestnut Street, Philadelphia PA 1906, USA

British Library Cataloguing in Publication Data
A catalogue record for this book is available from the British Library.

ISBN: 1 86156 206 3

Printed and bound in the UK by Athenaeum Press Ltd,
Gateshead, Tyne & Wear

Contents

Foreword

Human rights violations have a negative impact on health. It is therefore inconceivable to separate health and human rights and they need to be integrated into all aspects of health care including policy, programme planning, implementation, monitoring and evaluation.

(International Council of Nurses,
Human Rights and Health 99/8)

Why are human rights so important in the twenty-first century? Why is it that they feel so new for many nurses in the context of health? Just because human rights are now set out in an Act of Parliament, does this mean that its interpretation in relation to health issues can only be done by lawyers? How can nurses ensure a vital contribution in shaping the future of healthcare provision in the United Kingdom?

Learning about human rights has been likened to going to the dentist. It has got to be done, but somehow it seems easier to put it off. However, the importance of human rights in the twenty-first century is so fundamental to healthcare that ignorance is simply not an option for any nurse in the European Union.

The impact of the Human Rights Act 1998, which came into effect in October 2000, will be profound in health. It will alter the fundamental relationship that nurses have with patients and clients. The way that the government decides issues about the future development of healthcare will have to take account of the Act. All regulatory bodies involved with health will be affected, including the bodies that regulate the professions in health, the establishments in health and the services in health. Working relationships between those involved in health and social care will change as a result of the legislation. The media, of course, will be aware of human rights as a new angle to pursue in reporting on health issues.

This book aims to explain the Human Rights Act 1998 in a way that is accessible to all nurses in the United Kingdom. In addition, it assesses the impact of human rights on the various people and organizations that will be applying these new rights in all areas of health.

I am happy to commend this timely book as a valuable resource to all health professionals as they adapt policy and practice to conform to the important human rights principles required by contemporary legislation.

Baroness Caroline Cox

Introduction

The Human Rights Act, which received Royal Assent in 1998, came into force in October 2000. United Kingdom law will make what has been described by some as the most important change to individual rights since the Magna Carta. The Act will allow people to claim their rights under the European Convention of Human Rights in the UK courts and tribunals, instead of having to go to the European Court of Human Rights in Strasbourg. The Human Rights Act recognizes that all individuals have certain minimum and fundamental human rights. It represents a shift in previous constitutional thinking, which implied that individuals could do as they liked, unless Parliament or common law said they could not.

It is anticipated that people will gradually become more aware of their rights although it is not possible to predict the Act's impact with any certainty. One can only surmise that the increase in litigation, which has been experienced in other countries that have incorporated the Convention into domestic law, will be mirrored in the UK.

The new Act protects human rights under three broad categories:

1. Fundamental rights – for example, the right to life and the right not to be subjected to torture.
2. Procedural rights – such as the right to a fair trial and a fair hearing.
3. Qualified rights – such as freedom of expression and the right to freedom of association.

Many terms are not precise, so the Act does not enshrine many specific rights as such. It simply gives a context in which the courts must act.

The 'right to health' was first recognized as a fundamental right in 1946 when the constitution of the World Health Organization was adopted at the International Health Conference held in New York and supported by 61 states. These rights are now enshrined in several international treaties prepared by the World Health Organization (WHO) and including the *Universal Declaration of Human Rights* (UDHR).

Awareness of the Human Rights Act and its implications are crucial for nurses. They are often at the forefront of critical decisions and procedures and are able to see the immediate effects on patients and their relatives. Although only an individual can actually bring a case, nurses may be able to advise individuals how to proceed if necessary. More positively, an awareness of human rights issues may lead to a review of policies and protocols before a problem arises.

This book is mainly directed at understanding the impact that the Human Rights Act can be expected to make on healthcare. It attempts to put human rights into context by exploring the evolution of rights, international human rights, and more specifically human rights as they might affect nursing.

Christine Hancock
General Secretary
Royal College of Nursing

Chapter 1
Background to
Human Rights

Context and general importance

Human rights are now of tremendous importance for nurses. This chapter sets out the background of the development of rights in the United Kingdom and reviews some international approaches to human rights.

The theory of human rights is one thing: putting it into practice is another. It is important to have a broad understanding of the development of rights and the reasons for this. The broad context is defined in language and terms that are readily understood.

Evolution of rights

The concept of human rights is fairly new, but the concept of rights, particularly moral rights, stretches back to the earliest civilizations. Sophocles and Plato discussed the basis on which societies could exist with systems of rights. The relationship between governments and citizens was given legal status in England with the signing of the Magna Carta in 1215. This was a written contract between the King and his subjects and between his descendants and their descendants 'forever'. The Magna Carta guaranteed the freedom of the Church from royal interference; protected the property and inheritance rights of children and widows; limited taxes; set up courts to deal with criminal and civil issues; and stated that punishment should fit the crime. It forbade officials to steal from citizens, noblemen or free-born commoners, and forbade bribery of judges and other legal authorities. It also set out concepts of due process for the courts. More than five centuries later, the French *Declaration of the Rights of Man and the Citizen* in 1789 arose during a bloody revolution, which

1

saw the overthrow of the system in which the monarch was considered to be the basis through which all law was made.

Within the history of the development of human rights, it is possible to trace distinct forms of thinking over the past three centuries.

Freedom and first generation human rights

John Stuart Mill, writing in the nineteenth century, proposed a structure of libertarianism that was ground breaking in its day. He advocated that the value of freedom depends on the use to which it is put. The purpose of human rights in this context was to enhance dignity and to ensure the free development of personalities.

Mill's theories were based on a belief that the ultimate historical purpose of human rights is to foster and nurture a person's individual autonomy. In this model of human rights, the most fundamental right was the freedom of choice, and the model's purpose was to keep the state from interfering with the private freedom of the individual. Discussions at that time looked at the position of those who were unable to have this freedom of choice. Mill's famous remark 'the man who is hungry is not free, but the slave with a full belly is still a slave' created a wide debate about the value of having these rights if there was a section of society that was not able to exercise them.

Equality and second generation human rights

The development of Mill's model led to conflict in the twentieth century as emerging thinking proposed that there had to be a bridge between unlimited liberty and social justice. The debate led to recognition that there was value in using the state as a safety net in order to ensure equality. This in turn created the social acceptance for the introduction of the concept of the welfare state.

In contrast to the first generation human rights, the second generation human rights were concerned with extensive state interference to ensure social and economic equality. It can be seen from this that libertarianism and social equality are in fundamental conflict with each other. The balance needed to limit rights, which either conflict with each other or produce unwelcome effects, continues to exercise those involved in moral philosophy.

Global solidarity and third generation human rights

This is the newest form of human right and has arisen during the twentieth century. It is a model of human rights influenced by the global context and proposes that there should be a global reallocation of resources to ensure that the poorest countries of the world can afford to build the institutions necessary to protect human rights. However, the challenge of this model is that, in order to work, human rights must be inherently universal. They are supposed to belong to every individual regardless of gender, age, nationality, ethnic origin or culture. Before this third generation of human rights, it was easy to see that moral rights could be defined by those practices deemed unacceptable by a society. Arranged marriages, child labour, female circumcision, are all practices that do not fit the Western model of human rights, but which are an inherent part of other cultures. However, all these examples of cultural practice are forbidden by the *UN Universal Declaration of Human Rights* 1948. It might be argued that this is a form of moral imperialism that does not achieve the aim of global rights for all.

How do we develop a fourth generation of human rights?

It has been argued that wealth and better education are the main reasons why nations can adopt and give credence to human rights, and that to impose a system of Western ideals on others is to be naïve. Combating the poverty or attempting even to sustain democratic elections is such a struggle for many countries that a desire for them to achieve consistent human rights is too difficult. It may be more effective to adopt a piecemeal approach to these issues of fundamental human rights by encouraging other countries to change their approaches bit by bit, starting for example, with a prohibition on torture. An *Economist* leader (12 April 1997) urged development of human rights by continued piecemeal pressure: 'Pressure for human rights discomforts oppressors, encourages their victims and, in the long run, makes the world safer.'

Written codes of human rights: friend or foe?

One of the principal disadvantages of making a written code for human rights is that it then becomes fixed. It reflects the social thinking at the time it was written and therefore may become inflexible against changes in public perception over the years. The principles that led John Stuart Mill to set out a thesis on personal freedom were not translated into an Act of Parliament. If they had been, what would be the effect every time that Parliament wanted to change its mind about a newer model of human rights? It might be particularly unsettling for a nation to find that the principles that were held to sum up the values of their grandparents were considered to be of little relevance a mere two generations later. In the United Kingdom, for example, the death penalty was socially acceptable until half a century ago, with the last two people being hanged in August 1964. The death penalty continues to be used in many parts of the United States of America. Public opinion towards the death penalty is therefore different even in parts of the Western world.

Similar issues apply to the moral codes in religion. Where there are written texts, these cannot be rewritten in the same way as an Act of Parliament, which can be repealed entirely if it is no longer appropriate. Many theologians consider the wording of texts such as the Bible and the Koran to interpret and reinterpret the principles that are set out in these moral codes. The governing body for Jehovah's Witnesses reconsidered its written beliefs and agreed in June 2000 that, in certain circumstances, it is now possible for followers to have blood transfusions.

However, the pace at which thinking on a global scale is moving means that some flexibility for shaping human rights is needed. The current debate asks how it can be possible for codes of human rights to contain the flexibility needed to ensure that they last and that they retain public confidence.

Activity 1

Think of one aspect of health that has changed over the past 100 years.

Discussion points

- What were the values that were associated with it at that time?
- What are the values that are now associated with this change?

International human rights

The United Nations and human rights

The United Nations was established at the end of the Second World War in 1945. Human rights were a preoccupation of the new United

Nations such that, only three years later, the UN published a *Universal Declaration of Human Rights* to promote and protect human rights in the aftermath of the war. Article 1 of this Declaration states: 'all human beings are born free and equal in dignity and rights. They are endowed with reason and conscience and should act towards one another in a spirit of brotherhood.'

The Declaration sets out the belief that respect for human rights and human dignity 'is the foundation of freedom, justice and peace in the world'. Although it is not legally binding, many countries have incorporated the provisions into their laws and constitutions. International covenants and conventions have the force of law for the states that ratify them. The *International Covenant on Economic, Social and Cultural Rights* and the *International Covenant on Civil and Political Rights* are legally binding human rights agreements. Both were adopted by the UN General Assembly in 1966 and entered into force 10 years later, making many of the provisions of the *Universal Declaration of Human Rights* effectively binding.

The Commission on Human Rights is the main policy-making body dealing with human rights issues at the United Nations. It is made up of 53 member governments and prepares studies, makes recommendations and drafts international human rights conventions and declarations. It also investigates allegations of human rights violations and handles communications relating to them.

The Centre for Human Rights, which is part of the UN Secretariat in Geneva, operates a 24-hour fax 'hotline' for victims of human rights violations, their relatives and non-governmental organizations. It allows the Centre for Human Rights to react rapidly to human rights emergencies. The impact of the United Nations on human rights has been significant and has led to concrete results, such as the suspension of executions, release of detainees and medical treatment for prisoners, as well as changes in the domestic legal system of states who are party to human rights instruments. The post of High Commissioner for Human Rights was established in December 1993. This UN official has the principal responsibility for human rights activities, including promoting and protecting human rights for all and maintaining a continuing dialogue with Member states. It is part of the remit of the Centre for Human Rights to implement the policies proposed by the High Commissioner.

International human rights and health

There is no single source of health rights in international law, but many of the Conventions include them. Article 25 of the *UN Universal Declaration of Human Rights* establishes the overriding principle: 'Everyone has the right to a standard of living adequate for the health and well-being of himself and his family, including food, clothing, housing and medical care and necessary social services.' This aims to guarantee the preconditions of good health, including the availability of health services.

Different countries have sought to recognize basic rights, such as the right to health, in different ways. Canada has a system that protects human rights while preserving the sovereignty of Parliament. If there is a conflict between the rights set out in the Canadian Charter and other legislation, the Charter rights are given precedence. The offending legislation is not struck out but it is made clear that the offending part of the Act is no longer applicable. Parliament then has the opportunity to amend the legislation to comply with the Charter.

In New Zealand any conflict between the rights and legislation is resolved in favour of the legislation. The National Council for Civil Liberties has pointed out that in such a system, where the individual or group of people complaining that their rights had been infringed were regarded as an unpopular group, it may mean that Parliament never gets round to amending the legislation.

The World Health Organization's (WHO) current health policy 'Health for all - towards the 21st century' is designed to meet future health challenges and has been developed by WHO in consultation with its national and international partners. WHO seeks the highest attainable standard of health as one of the fundamental rights of every human being (WHO 1998).

WHO is a specialized agency of the United Nations with 191 member states. Its main functions are to give world-wide guidance in the field of health, set global standards for health, strengthen national health programmes in co-operation with governments and to develop health technology, information and standards.

The UK has also signed up to the European Social Charter 1961 which has been produced by the Council of Europe. At a meeting in Rome 1990, ministers agreed that the Social Charter is 'a fundamental document enshrining social and civic rights' and that 'it is important to stress the inseparable nature of human, civil political, social, economic and cultural rights' (ESC1998). Article 13 of this Charter commits the UK authorities to ensure that necessary care is provided for those who are sick and without adequate resources to secure such assistance for themselves. While this Charter does not have the same legal force as the Human Rights Act 1998, it may have some impact on interpretation and might produce action in individual cases.

Human rights law has also recognized that the health rights for some specific groups may need special attention. The United Nations Convention on the Rights of the Child 1990 contains both a general statement on children's health rights and a series of specific commitments.

Human rights and nurses

The International Council of Nurses

The International Council of Nurses (ICN) is a federation of more than 120 national nurses' associations representing millions of nurses world-wide. Operated by nurses for nurses, the ICN is the international voice of nursing and works to ensure quality care for all and sound health policies globally. The ICN has published a statement of human rights and health (see Appendix 3), which requires nurses to take account of the following:

> National nurses' associations, individual nurses and other health care providers must play a leading role in strengthening the vital link between health and human rights and thereby contribute to prevention of disease and enhance equitable access to health care.

(ICN/99/8)

The United Kingdom Central Council for Nursing, Midwifery and Health Visiting

The UKCC is the regulatory body for nurses, midwives and health visitors. It produces a Code of Conduct, which sets out the basic principles that must be followed by nurses and midwives. When a complaint is made that a nurse or midwife has not followed this Code of Conduct, the UKCC has a range of sanctions that can be imposed on the individual nurse or midwife, including the most serious measure of removing the nurse or midwife from the register. Although the Code of Conduct does not mention human rights, the UKCC is obliged to follow the law. The Human Rights Act 1998 therefore will have to be taken into account in all existing and future guidance given by the UKCC, including the matters contained in the Code of Conduct. The UKCC, as the regulatory body, has the authority to alter the Code of Conduct and to introduce new principles that all nurses and midwives need to follow.

Activity 2

Look at the UKCC Code of Conduct.

Discussion point

- Do you think there are any principles that could be added to the Code which specifically deal with human rights?

Chapter 2
The European
Convention on
Human Rights

History of the Council of Europe

The threat to fundamental human rights and to political freedom following the ending of the Second World War led many countries in Europe to take a new look at the way in which international law was formulated. Human rights had been a matter between individual countries and their citizens. Other countries did not interfere with those arrangements unless their own citizens were under threat. By the late 1940s, many countries in Europe agreed that the rights of citizens might require protection against their own state. A collective guarantee for fundamental human rights was seen as a way of ensuring wider consistency and protection of the citizens of a number of different states.

The Council of Europe

On 5 May 1949, the Council of Europe was founded and the member states drafted the Convention for the Protection of Human Rights and Fundamental Freedoms of 4 November 1950. This is now what is generally known as the European Convention on Human Rights.

The Council of Europe is an organization devoted to the principles of democracy, the rule of law and respect for human rights. Its aim is to 'achieve a greater unity between its Members for the purpose of safeguarding and realising the ideals and principles which are their common heritage and facilitating their economic and social progress' (Article 1 of the Statute of the Council of Europe 1949). The Council elects a Secretary-General as its senior official for a period of five years.

9

The European Union

The Council of Europe should not be confused with the European Union (EU). The EU is a union of 15 independent states based on the European Communities and founded to enhance political, economic and social co-operation. The EU, which was formerly known as the European Community (EC) or European Economic Community (EEC), was founded on 1 November 1993. The European Court of Justice at Luxembourg is the court that has been set up to work out how best to interpret European Union law. It will take the Convention on Human Rights into account but it is not required to regard the Convention as a source of EU law. It has in the past even interpreted provisions of the Convention contrary to the interpretations made by the European Court on Human Rights.

The European Convention of Human Rights

The Convention, which came into effect on 4 November 1950, is an agreement by which member states of the Council of Europe undertake to secure certain fundamental human rights. The Convention itself consists of Articles and Protocols. Articles 2–18 were not considered to cover all the issues needed as time went by, and so further Protocols were added at different times. Protocols 1,4,6 and 7 have been incorporated in the Convention along with the original Articles.

- Articles 2–18 set out the freedoms and liberties.
- Articles 19–51 deal with the establishment of the European Court of Human Rights and the processes for dealing with allegations of violations against the Convention.
- Articles 52–59 deal with miscellaneous items.
- Protocol 1 has six Articles, which deal with property and education rights, and came into effect on 20 March 1952.
- Protocol 4 has seven Articles, which deal with freedom of movement, and came into effect on 16 September 1963.
- Protocol 6 has nine Articles, which deal with the death penalty, and came into effect on 28 April 1983.

The member states of the Council of Europe: who has signed what

As of June 2000, 41 countries have signed up to the Convention. These member states of the Council of Europe have signed up to the rights and freedoms in the Articles, but not all of them have signed up to all the further Protocols. The UK, for example, was the first country to ratify the Convention and signed up to the Convention on 3 September 1953 as well as Protocol 1, but did not sign up to Protocols 4 or 6. Iceland however, has signed up to the Convention and all the Protocols. In signing up to the Convention, these countries have accepted the jurisdiction of the European Court of Human Rights and the right of individual petition.

Some member states have lodged reservations or derogations that may affect the protection of certain rights and freedoms. It is therefore important that anyone making an application to the Commission with a complaint that a right or freedom has not been upheld, is sure that the member state has not limited itself in this way. The UK, for example, lodged reservations in 1953 when it became a signatory to Protocol 1, which provides a right to education. The UK will only be bound by this provision where it is compatible with the provision of efficient instruction. A derogation was lodged by the UK to Article 5(3) in connection with the prompt trial of those arrested in Northern Ireland.

Where a person wanted to make a complaint about health, it would be necessary for their lawyers to ensure that the UK had signed up to a particular aspect of the Convention before making that claim.

The European Commission of Human Rights

The European Commission of Human Rights is an independent international body set up under the European Convention of Human Rights. Member states of the Council of Europe agree to basic provisions of human rights. Each country signing up to the Convention has one member on the Commission. The members of the Commission are independent of governments and do not have any duty to represent their country on the Commission.

Who can make a complaint to the Commission?

The Commission can receive complaints that a member state has violated rights or freedoms recognized under the Convention from an individual, groups of persons, or non-governmental organizations. The person making the complaint must claim that a member state has, *to their personal detriment*, violated one of the freedoms or rights in the Convention or one of the Protocols. The Commission cannot receive complaints on behalf of third parties or complaints of a general nature. In this respect, the Commission acts no differently from the way that courts and tribunals operate in the UK. Although a group of people may find that there is a fault in the way that health services are being provided, it is necessary for an individual to make a claim that he or she has personally been affected before any claim that the Convention has been violated can be made.

The Commission can only deal with complaints about matters that are the responsibility of a public authority. These may include courts, tribunals or administrative bodies. The Commission cannot deal with complaints against private persons or organizations. It is not possible, therefore, for the Commission to deal with complaints about neighbours or local sports clubs that are not the responsibility of a public authority.

What can the Commission do?

The Commission cannot intervene directly with the national authorities concerned on behalf of a complainant. However, if the matter seems to be urgent, the Commission may suggest some interim steps that could be taken which are in the interests of the parties. The Commission is not a court of appeal from national court decisions and cannot overturn the decisions made by the courts or tribunals.

When do you make a complaint to the Commission?

It is necessary to show the Commission that the person making the complaint has already used all the available means in the courts in their own country to try and resolve the problem. In England and Wales this will involve a hearing at the House of Lords, the Judicial Committee of the Privy Council or the Courts-Martial Appeal Court before making a complaint to the Commission. In Scotland, the highest domestic court is the High Court of Justiciary or the Court of Session and in Northern Ireland the highest domestic court is the Court of Appeal.

As set out in Article 26 of the European Convention of Human Rights, there is a short and fixed period of only six months to make a complaint to the Commission from the date that the final domestic court made its order. This time limit is strictly observed. Any application outside the six months will simply be returned to the complainant.

How do you make a complaint to the Commission?

Very simply, you write a letter. The letter must contain the following:

- an outline of the complaint,
- an indication of the rights or freedoms that are alleged to have been violated,

- a list of the remedies that have been tried in the member state,
- a list of the official decisions that have been made by the courts, with dates and details of the decisions.

Once the Commission has the letter, the Secretary to the Commission will reply and may ask for more information about the case. The Secretary may also give information about the way that the Commission has dealt with similar claims in the past. The Secretary cannot give advice about the law or the current policy in the member state concerned, but this remains a fairly informal exchange of information at this stage. If the letter has been submitted outside the time limit, for example, or the member state is not a signatory to the particular freedom being complained about, the Secretary will notify the complainant that the matter cannot proceed.

Once the Secretary is satisfied that there is sufficient documentation about the case, the matter is passed to the Commission. All these initial stages are in writing and are private. It is not possible to see the correspondence between the complainant and the Secretary at this stage. In this respect, the application is different from starting court proceedings where the documentation is a matter of public record.

What does the Commission do?

The Commission makes a decision about the admissibility of the application and seeks views from both the member state and the complainant. Once the Commission decides to admit an application it is required under Article 28 of the Convention to try and secure a settlement between the parties, the applicant and the state. If this succeeds, it is known as a 'friendly settlement'. Otherwise the Commission draws up a Report, which remains confidential, and which is sent to the Committee of Ministers of the Council of Europe and the parties. A three-month period then runs during which the case is referred to the European Court of Human Rights.

The European Court of Human Rights

The European Court of Human Rights is based in Strasbourg. All hearings are in public. The Court gives a judgment in which it decides whether or not a violation of the Convention has taken place. The Court's decision is final and is binding on the country concerned. The remedy for the complainant is an order of compensation and reimbursement of legal costs.

However, the decisions made by the Court have no legal precedent. In theory they are limited to their own facts. In practice, all countries are bound by the principles arising from a judgment. The country involved in the case may need to take steps to change its domestic law or administrative procedures as a result of the Court's decision. Other countries may want to consider whether the judgment has an effect on their own law.

There are two doctrines that are used by the European Court of Human Rights: margin of appreciation and principle of proportionality.

Margin of appreciation

The Court is international in its jurisdiction and so it allows the state a margin of appreciation. This means that it allows a measure of discretion in its action, which reflects the Court's recognition that it needs to be sensitive to the totality of the culture of the state. The interpretation of the Convention should, if possible, reflect widespread European practice.

Principle of proportionality

This doctrine means that the Court balances the interests of the community with the rights of the individual. The action must be no more than is required to address a 'pressing social need' (*Soering* v *United Kingdom* (1989) 11 EHRR 439). The action required by the state must affect the freedom of the individual as little as possible. There must be consistency in the way that the state carries out its actions.

Remedies

What happens if a person is successful in their claim that a human right has been violated? The Court can order that compensation is paid to the individual and can award them their legal costs of bringing the case. More importantly, however, from a health perspective is that a ruling in favour of the applicant against the current system in their country is likely to have a direct effect on the way that all future policy is developed in that area. As a result, many people take a case to the Commission more on a point of principle than to obtain compensation. Where the European Court of Human Rights determines the way that a country operates a policy or a procedure, the country will have to look for practical ways of changing the system to bring it in line with the judgment.

Chapter 3
The Human Rights
Act 1998:
How Does it Work?

How law is made in the United Kingdom

Legislation

An Act of Parliament sets out the law in a formal document. Examples of statutes are the Children Act 1989, the Human Embryology and Fertilisation Act 1990, the Access to Medical Records Act 1990 and the Medicinal Products – Prescription by Nurses etc Act 1992. Each Act of Parliament follows a formal and detailed procedure of debate and voting in the House of Commons and the House of Lords. Statutes form a body of law that sets out in detail how individuals must act. If someone fails to act in accordance with any part of a statute, a criminal penalty may be imposed. For example, a driver who is found with excess alcohol in his blood may be charged with a criminal offence under the Road Traffic Acts, which set out the relevant legal limits.

Delegated or secondary legislation allows for more detailed statutory rules to be drawn up without requiring debating time in the House of Commons. These are known as statutory instruments. The Nursing, Midwives and Health Visitors Act 1997 creates a legal duty for the United Kingdom Central Council for Nursing, Midwifery and Health Visiting (UKCC) to hold professional conduct hearings into allegations of improper conduct on the part of a nurse. The rules that govern the conduct hearing itself are provided in a statutory instrument (The Nurses, Midwives and Health Visitors Rules 1993). The effect of this statutory instrument is to oblige the UKCC to follow a certain procedure in its investigations and hearings of these matters.

A further source of legislation comes from Europe, which requires member states to implement Community law through their own Acts of Parliament. European legislation, which is also known as European Directives, encompasses a variety of issues, including the 1990 European Directive (90/269/EEC) on the manual handling of loads and Directive 92/85/EEC on the protection of the rights of pregnant workers.

Common law

Where no legislation exists to determine the law on a particular subject, common law will be used. Common law is made by judges who sit in court and determine how a legal dispute between two or more parties is to be resolved. The law relating to negligence, for example, is not defined in a statute, but has evolved over time through various court decisions. These decisions form a body of law. Patients who allege that negligent treatment has led to injury will have their disputes heard in court, and the legal principles that apply will be those of the common law of negligence.

Case law can also be used to interpret the law in the statutes of both Acts of Parliament and Statutory Instruments. In the case of *R* v *Coughlan ex parte North and East Devon Health Authority* (*Times Law Report*, 20 July 1999), the Court of Appeal found that where the Health Authority was planning to charge for nursing services in a nursing home, this was unlawful and outside the powers contained in the National Assistance Act 1948. The judgment interpreted the wording of a section in that Act, which is now the basis on which that particular section has to be understood. The common law has defined the way that legislation is used.

The Human Rights Act 1998

The Human Rights Act 1998 came into effect in England, Northern Ireland and Wales on 2 October 2000. It became effective in Scotland on 1 July 1999. Why the delay between the Act being made and the Act becoming effective? The answer is simple: the Human Rights Act will affect every area of law concerning the individual. The Convention will not simply be bolted on to UK law: it will instead mean that a fundamentally different approach to the interpretation of statute and case law will take place. Because this change is so extreme, all public bodies and institutions needed time to conduct an audit of their working practices and to have training so that as soon as the Act came into force they would be able to implement the provisions.

The Lord Chancellor has set aside at least £4.5 million as specific funding to deal with the cost of training judges, magistrates and tribunal chairmen in using the Human Rights Act. A further £60 million has been earmarked for legal aid cases that are likely to contain points about the Human Rights Act (Lord Chancellor's media briefing, November 1998).

The UK had not previously incorporated the Convention into its own law and this has meant that anyone who has wanted to make a claim that a right had been violated has had no other option but to take that claim to the European Court of Human Rights. The courts in the UK have simply lacked the authority to consider the articles of the Convention until now. As a result, the UK has had almost as many referrals claiming breach of human rights as Turkey. That situation has now changed as the courts in the UK can and must consider claims about the Convention rights whenever asked to do so. It should also avoid the delay that has exasperated many claimants who have waited several years to have their cases heard in Europe.

The rights in the Convention are about principles. This differs from UK legislation, which is practical and specific in detail, although again it seems to be the case that recent legislation is framed in governing duties; the Health Act 1999, for example, creates a duty for health authorities to consider partnership arrangements, with detailed government guidance to follow about how the partnership arrangements are to take place. The right to life, and the right not to be tortured are fundamental principles, but they are capable of subjective judgements of value and therefore require that the judge apply subjective ideas and opinions rather than the technical interpretation of a line or a section in an Act.

The Human Rights Act 1998 means that any legislation which exists in the UK must now be considered in the light of the Convention and 'read and given effect in a way which is compatible with the Convention rights' (s. 3(1)).

To what extent will the decisions about social policy be handed over to the courts? This difficulty was recognized at the time the Act was passed. In a case concerning the rights of unmarried fathers to have parental responsibility for their children, Mrs Justice Hale said 'there are real dangers in attempting to conduct debates about social policy through the medium of the courts. They are for the resolution through the democratic rather than the judicial process' (*Re W* v *Re B (Child Abduction –Unmarried Father)* [1998] 2 FLR 146). Even at this stage, the judges were realizing the responsibility that has been passed on to them.

Public authorities

Section 6 of the Act says that 'It is unlawful for a public authority to act in a way which is incompatible with a Convention right'.

The definition of public authority is very wide. It includes those bodies where all or any of its functions are functions of a public nature (s. 6 (3)). This will include central government, executive agencies, local government, the police, immigration services and prisons. The Houses of Parliament are excluded from being a public authority. It also includes the NHS and social services as well as all their agencies. It includes the courts and all tribunals.

The Act will make it unlawful for public authorities to act in ways that are incompatible with the Convention. The Lord Chancellor has commented that the definition of public authority has deliberately been left broadly drawn in order to provide as much protection as possible for individuals against the state. The UK Courts will have the authority and the duty to consider the effects of each of the articles in the Human Rights Act where they are put forward by the claimant. 'The Human Rights Act, for example, will lead the courts to exercise a more intensive form of scrutiny over government and public authorities' (Lord Chancellor, Press release, 5 July 1999).

The impact of the Human Rights Act will be that all public authorities will have to make human rights a central part of the development of its functions. As Aisling Reidy points out (unpublished discussion paper Nuffield Trust 1999) 'the structure of the Human Rights Act in placing statutory obligations on public authorities to be human rights compliant, by virtue of sections 3 and 6, promotes the development of best practice rather than a risk management approach.'

Some private bodies can be considered to be public authorities where they exercise public functions. Companies that undertake functions that were previously undertaken by the public sector will be 'public authorities' to the extent that they are carrying out activities that would otherwise be provided by the state. This leaves nursing homes in a very complex situation. They could find themselves in the position of fulfilling both a public function if they undertake caring for patients on behalf of the NHS or social services and private functions if they care for patients on an independent basis. Where they fulfil a public function, they will be a public authority and accountable under the Human Rights Act. Regulatory bodies, some charities and other organisations who carry out public functions will also fall within this category of public authority.

It may be possible for a person to claim that the courts have a positive obligation to give them legal protection from situations such as press intrusion. It is also possible to argue that the Press Complaints Commission is a public authority, in order to push for stronger sanctions against newspapers who infringe its Code of Practice.

Section 6 provides that it is unlawful for a public authority to act in a way that is incompatible with a Convention right unless, as a result of primary legislation, the authority could not have acted differently. So where a court gives effect to European Union law in a way that conflicts with the Convention the court will be able to argue that it could not have acted differently.

Victims: the new applicants

Only a person who is or would be a 'victim' of an action by a public authority can make a complaint under the Act. This means that a challenge to the Convention must be brought by a person affected by the Article; it cannot be brought by a person who wants the law changed for its own sake. Where a group of nurses wish to bring a case that a right has been broken, this is allowed under the Act as long as the nurses are directly affected by the Article. They cannot bring the case on behalf of a patient.

For example, if some nurses were concerned that the rights of patients were being affected in a mixed sex ward, they would not be able to bring a claim on behalf of patients generally. It would have to be one or more patients that brought the claim as victims under the Act. Nurses would be able to support the claim that the rights had been broken, either by giving factual evidence or expert evidence. In this way, the court would be made aware of nursing practice in a particular area.

Interpretative obligation

Section 3 introduces a new obligation of interpretation. There has never been such a principle before. It requires that where a Court finds that some existing legislation is at odds with the Convention rights, it may make a declaration that either the primary legislation or the secondary legislation is incompatible with those rights. The Courts that can carry out such a review are:

- the House of Lords
- the Judicial Committee of the Privy Council
- The Courts-Martial Appeal Court
- The High Court of Justiciary (Scotland)
- The High Court
- The Court of Appeal

This 'declaration of incompatibility' could have tremendous impact. It does not affect the legal nature of the legislation in question. Section 10 allows ministers substantial powers to make amendments to legislation where it has been subject to a declaration of incompatibility or where the European Court of Human Rights has declared that there is a conflict. This power means that the minister would be able to bypass the normal legislative process and make amendments by order, even where this would entail the repeal of relevant provisions or of entire pieces of primary legislation.

Absolute rights

Some of the Articles contain absolute rights, which are not qualified in any way. For example, Article 3 contains an absolute right not to be subjected to degrading treatment. The lack of any qualification allowing this type of activity to take place in certain circumstances means that it will be easier, in health-related issues, for people to consider whether their rights have been violated. This will be particularly so in health, where any activity that a patient feels is degrading could be considered. It has been of particular importance in mental health.

Qualified rights

Many of the rights in the Convention are qualified and are therefore diluted to some extent (see Appendix 2). These qualifications are broad in nature, and mean that the headline right is to be interpreted by other considerations. The qualifications in the Act are: whether the matter is in the interests of national security or public interest, for the prevention of crime, or the protection of health or morals or the rights and freedoms of others. For example, the right to private life is subject to limitations, such as the protection of health and the prevention of crime.

Positive and negative obligations

The language in the Convention means that the government is required in some of the Articles to take positive steps to ensure that some of the rights and freedoms are promoted. The positive obligations in Article 2 (right to life), Article 3 (freedom from degrading behaviour) and Article 8 (right to privacy) mean that the government cannot simply fulfil its obligations passively. The government has to take positive steps to ensure that these rights are given teeth and that they are promoted.

Procedures for challenge

Where an action is brought against a public authority, the Act allows a period of one year from the date of the alleged breach for this to be taken to court. For example, where a patient or a client believes that being treated on a mixed sex ward is outside the rights contained in the Act, they have one year from the date of that treatment to get legal advice and begin court proceedings.

Nurses may be asked by the patient's representative to confirm the nature of the treatment so that the facts of the case can be confirmed. In most cases brought under the European Convention of Human Rights, there is usually no dispute about what happened and the bulk of the legal argument is centred on whether those facts can be interpreted to be a violation of the rights in the Convention. In such cases, therefore, the nurse may want to contact her professional organization for advice. Generally, her manager should be informed so that if there is contact with the patient's solicitor or representative to confirm the facts, that can be done in a way that is least stressful for everyone concerned.

Where the patient does take the case to court, the judge will have a duty to consider the facts, hear the arguments from both sides about whether it is a violation of a particular right, and then decide if indeed such a violation has taken place. The nurse may be called to confirm the facts and, if so, it would be advisable for her to have a representative with her to explain the court etiquette and procedure.

At the end of the hearing, if the patient has won his or her argument, that case will be a precedent for anyone else in a similar situation. They would be able to rely on that judgment to persuade the public authority to change its procedures or treatment for them.

Chapter 4
The Articles and Protocols of the Human Rights Act 1998

This chapter outlines the Articles and Protocols of the Human Rights Act 1998. The full Act can be found in Appendix 1 and a further summary of these Articles can be found in Appendix 2.

Article 1: Obligation to secure rights and freedoms

> The High Contracting Parties shall secure to everyone within their jurisdiction the rights and freedoms defined in Section 1 of this Convention.

The Convention secures certain rights and freedoms. Civil and political rights are covered in the Convention and provide protection against executive action. Where social and economic rights exist in the United Nations Declaration, they appear as standards to be attained, depending on the level of economic development. Social and economic rights are not covered in the Convention, so there is, for example, no right to basic health care. The Protocols begin to encroach on economic and social rights, so that Article 1 of the First Protocol protects property rights and Article 2 guarantees the right to education.

The importance of Article 1 of the Convention is that the rights contained in the rest of the Convention are not to be taken as standards to be achieved by the states; this Article transforms the declaration of the rights of the individual into a set of obligations to be followed.

23

There is a double responsibility that states have to adopt in relation to Article 1. On the one hand the states have to implement the Articles and the Protocols of the Convention and to ensure that there are systems in place for this. On the other hand, the states have to ensure that they themselves do not infringe the rights contained in the Articles and Protocols. Where this occurs, the state must provide a remedy for the wrong committed, whether that wrong was carried out by the state or by a private individual.

The UK government has ratified the Convention and has now incorporated this in the Human Rights Act 1998. The government therefore has to give effect to the Articles which give individuals rights and freedoms. This duty began in 1950. In any cases where the UK has been the subject of a case before the European Court of Human Rights, and has lost the case, it has taken steps to alter the offending action.

Article 2: Right to life

1. Everyone's right to life shall be protected by law. No one shall be deprived of his life intentionally save in the execution of a sentence of a court following his conviction of a crime for which this penalty is provided by law.
2. Deprivation of life shall not be regarded as inflicted in contravention of this Article when it results from the use of force which is no more than absolutely necessary:
   (a) in defence of any person from unlawful violence;
   (b) in order to effect a lawful arrest or to prevent the escape of a person lawfully detained;
   (c) in action lawfully taken for the purpose of quelling a riot or insurrection.

There are positive obligations to preserve life, but the language of this Article does not say that 'everyone has a right to life'. What this Article does is to guarantee the use of law to safeguard a right to life.

In *LCB* v *United Kingdom* (1998) 4 BHRC 421 the case concerned a child who was at risk of developing leukaemia from her father who had been exposed to radiation while working on Christmas Island. The Court accepted the principle that if the state knew or ought to have known of a particular life-threatening risk it should warn those affected. This suggests that the Article places a burden on health bodies to make the public aware of environmental risks.

Euthanasia and abortion are not automatically prohibited by this Article. In *X* v *United Kingdom* (1979) 19 DR 244, the abortion was allowed 'for the health of the mother'. However, in another case, *H* v *Norway* (1992) 73 DR 155, the Court found that Article 2 would protect the foetus in 'certain circumstances', although these are not specified. In the case of *Paton* v *United Kingdom* (1980) 3 EHRR 408 the rights of the father to prevent an abortion were not allowed to be used as a means of asserting protection of a right to life.

In *Widmer* v *Switzerland* Application No 20527/92, the Commission found that allowing a person to die by witholding treatment may be permitted. However, this distinction in law is based on the notion of passive acts (not having the treatment) and does not allow active acts (deliberately giving oneself the lethal injection). It is an accepted part of civil law that an adult of sound mind has full autonomy to decide not to have further treatment even where the outcome is that he or she will die. The reasons for refusal do not have to be rational.

Article 3: Prohibition of torture

No one shall be subjected to torture or to inhuman or degrading treatment or punishment.

This Article is not qualified and is one of the few Articles that does not have some 'let out' clause, which would allow for interpretation. It is an absolute right. However there have been a number of decisions made by the European Court of Human Rights that have set parameters on this right.

In a very early decision, the Court has set out its preferred definition of 'degrading'. In the *Greek case* (1969) 12 Yearbook 186–510, the Court held that treatment can only be degrading if it grossly humiliates the victim or drives him to act against his will or conscience.

It seems that a prisoner who has been detained can be force-fed and treated against his will. In *X* v *Germany* (1985) 7 EHRR 152, the Court found that a prisoner who was being force-fed was not subject to degrading treatment as this was 'solely in the best interests' of the prisoner 'with a view to securing his health and even saving his life'.

However, in *Tanko* v *Finland* 23634/94 (1994) unreported, the Court decided that a failure to provide proper medical treatment could be a breach of Article 3. It is not clear what would be covered by the phrase 'proper medical treatment'. It may cover matters such as inadequate pain relief, or being made to wait on a trolley in an accident and emergency department.

The Court also has used Article 3 to justify a failure to provide treatment under the NHS. In the case of *D* v *United Kingdom* (1994) 24 EHRR 423, the Court found that to send the man who had AIDS back to his home country of St Kitts where there was no provision for his treatment amounted to 'acute mental and physical suffering'.

The issue of informed consent to treatment for those suffering from mental illness will be important for the government to show that it has taken positive steps to avoid infringement of this Article.

The rights of children will be important under this Article. In one significant case, *A* v *United Kingdom* [1998] EHRLR 82, the Court found that the parental right to smack a child was not an appropriate exemption to this Article. The Court found that parental smacking was incompatible with the positive duty on the government to prevent degrading treatment. Treatment on babies and young children with drugs which have not been tested may also amount to a breach under Article 3.

Article 4: Prohibition of slavery and forced labour

1. No one shall be held in slavery or servitude.
2. No one shall be required to perform forced or compulsory labour.
3. For the purpose of this Article the term "forced or compulsory labour" shall not include:
   (a) any work required to be done in the ordinary course of detention imposed according to the provisions of Article 5 of this Convention or during conditional release from such detention;
   (b) any service of a military character or, in case of conscientious objectors in countries where they are recognised, service exacted instead of compulsory military service;
   (c) any service exacted in case of an emergency or calamity threatening the life or well-being of the community;
   (d) any work or service which forms part of normal civic obligations.

Article 4(1) indicates that slavery and servitude are matters of status. This status, which appears to imply an ongoing status, is forbidden absolutely. There are no exemptions to this. Article 4(2) places a different emphasis on the right protected and prohibits forced or compulsory labour. This is intended to protect those who are at liberty but who are coerced into forced labour for temporary periods of time. It implies that those who work in enforced labour on a permanent basis fall then into the provisions of Article 4(1). The provisions of Article 4(2) are limited by those forms of work or service expressly permitted under Article 4(3).

In the case of *Iverson* v *Norway* (1963) 6 Yearbook 278, a dentist challenged a law in Norway that required him to work for two years in the public dental service. The Commission found that the application was not admissible and the case did not go to the Court. The Commission found that the service 'was for a short period, provided favourable remuneration, did not involve any diversion from chosen professional work . . . and did not involve any discriminatory, arbitrary or punitive application'.

It is open to discussion whether matters like junior doctors' hours, which cannot be avoided by those wishing to study to qualify as a doctor, are in contravention of this Article. The compulsory element of trainee doctors to work hours well in excess of the norm could imply that a doctor could complain about this to the Commission. The government has said that it intends to reduce the hours but that this will take time.

This is one of the few Articles in the Convention that has a number of exemptions, but which does not contain an exemption 'for the protection of health'.

Article 5: Right to liberty and security

1. Everyone has the right to liberty and security of person. No one shall be deprived of his liberty save in the following cases and in accordance with a procedure prescribed by law:

   (a) the lawful detention of a person after conviction by a competent court;

   (b) the lawful arrest or detention of a person for non-compliance with the lawful order of a court or in order to secure the fulfilment of any obligation prescribed by law;

   (c) the lawful arrest or detention of a person effected for the purpose of bringing him before the competent legal authority on reasonable suspicion of having committed an offence or when it is reasonably considered necessary to prevent his committing an offence or fleeing after having done so;

   (d) the detention of a minor by lawful order for the purpose of educational supervision or his lawful detention for the purpose of bringing him before the competent legal authority;

   (e) the lawful detention of persons for the prevention of the spreading of infectious diseases, of persons of unsound mind, alcoholics or drug addicts or vagrants;

   (f) the lawful arrest or detention of a person to prevent his effecting an unauthorised entry into the country or of a person against whom action is being taken with a view to deportation or extradition.

2. Everyone who is arrested shall be informed promptly, in a language which he understands, of the reasons for his arrest and of any charge against him.

3. Everyone arrested or detained in accordance with the provisions of paragraph 1(c) of this Article shall be brought promptly before a judge or other officer authorised by law to exercise judicial power and shall be entitled to trial within a reasonable time or to release pending trial. Release may be conditioned by guarantees to appear for trial.

4. Everyone who is deprived of his liberty by arrest or detention shall be entitled to take proceedings by which the lawfulness of his detention shall be decided speedily by a

court and his release ordered if the detention is not lawful.
5. Everyone who has been the victim of arrest or detention in
   contravention of the provisions of this Article shall have an
   enforceable right to compensation.

This Article guarantees everyone the right to liberty and security of
the person.

A person who believes that they have been unlawfully detained
can apply under Article 5(4) for a review. This would apply to a
review by a mental health tribunal as suggested by the case of X v
United Kingdom (1982) 4 EHRR 188. The Court found that a review
after eight weeks was unlawful (*E* v *Norway* (1994) 17 EHRR 30) and
while this did not set a tariff, it would have been noted by the government in this country. As a result of this case, significant changes have
been made to the law in the UK about the review process.

Whether a person can be said to be 'detained' is a matter of
degree. The Court has found that it extends a secure hospital and a
psychiatric hospital (*Ashingdane* v *United Kingdom* (1985) 7 EHRR 528).
Detention can only be justified if it takes place in a hospital, clinic or
other 'appropriate institution authorised for the purpose'. In the case
of *Johnson* v *United Kingdom*, 27 October 1997, a person was kept in a
psychiatric setting even though he no longer suffered from a mental
illness while the authorities looked for a suitable hostel for him. The
Court found that his detention was an infringement of Article 5.

Article 6: Right to a fair trial

1. In the determination of his civil rights and obligations or of any criminal charge against him, everyone is entitled to a fair and public hearing within a reasonable time by an independent and impartial tribunal established by law. Judgment shall be pronounced publicly but the press and public may be excluded from all or part of the trial in the interest of morals, public order or national security in a democratic society, where the interests of juveniles or the protection of the private life of the parties so require, or to the extent strictly necessary in the opinion of the court in special circumstances where publicity would prejudice the interests of justice.
2. Everyone charged with a criminal offence shall be presumed innocent until proved guilty according to law.
3. Everyone charged with a criminal offence has the following minimum rights:
    (a) to be informed promptly, in a language which he understands and in detail, of the nature and cause of the accusation against him;
    (b) to have adequate time and facilities for the preparation of his defence;
    (c) to defend himself in person or through legal assistance of his own choosing or, if he has not sufficient means to pay for legal assistance, to be given it free when the interests of justice so require;
    (d) to examine or have examined witnesses against him and to obtain the attendance and examination of witnesses on his behalf under the same conditions as witnesses against him;
    (e) to have the free assistance of an interpreter if he cannot understand or speak the language used in court.

This is one of the most important rights in the Convention. It will have an impact on every tribunal in the UK. It provides that there must be a guarantee of a fair trial in any civil or criminal proceedings. It means that all regulatory bodies will need to make sure that their procedures are compatible with the Article, otherwise anyone affected would have the ability to challenge the procedure. In a case involving a doctor, the Court held that a nine-year delay in dealing with disciplinary matters against a doctor was in violation of this Article (*Darnell* v *United Kingdom* Series A no 272).

The NHS complaints procedures will be subject to the requirements of Article 6 and the NHS will have to ensure that the processes used at all levels of complaints handling are independent and impartial, particularly where a complaint about the provision of treatment is made. It will also be important that people being refused NHS treatment are given reasons for this which are compatible with Article 6.

In a case concerning a GP (*Trivedi* v *United Kingdom* (1997) EHRLR 521), the GP was convicted of theft for claiming payments for visits to a patient which had not been made. The patient made statements about the extent of the visits but his illness meant that he was unable to give evidence at the trial. The judge took the statements and used these in the trial leading to the GP's conviction. The GP took his case to the European Court of Human Rights claiming that there had been a breach of Article 6(3) in that he had been unable to challenge the patient. His case failed. The Court found that the judge had made extensive investigations into the patient's condition and that the judge was also able to rely on prescription sheets written by the GP, which supported the patient's statement.

Article 7: No punishment without law

1. No one shall be held guilty of any criminal offence on account of any act or omission which did not constitute a criminal offence under national or international law at the time when it was committed. Nor shall a heavier penalty be imposed than the one that was applicable at the time the criminal offence was committed.
2. This Article shall not prejudice the trial and punishment of any person for any act or omission which, at the time when it was committed, was criminal according to the general principles of law recognised by civilised nations.

This Article means that no one can be found guilty of an offence when no criminal offence existed at that time. It binds the government in the way that it makes legislation, to ensure that it does not make an act unlawful in retrospect. It also binds the criminal courts from extending the scope of the criminal law by interpretation.

This Article does not appear to prohibit a second trial for the same offence, and it may be that the use of DNA testing technology may suggest that certain people could be tried again if new evidence becomes possible to obtain. Such a step would require the UK government to change its domestic law (commonly referred to as the law of 'double jeopardy') and if it did so, any second trial could only take place from the date of the new law.

The UK has been found to be in breach of this Article (*Welch* v *United Kingdom* (1995) 20 **EHRR** 247) when it tried to confiscate alleged proceeds of drugs trafficking under new regulations which came into force two months after Mr Welch was arrested.

The extent to which this Article has an impact on health law is unclear.

Article 8: Right to respect for private and family life

1. Everyone has the right to respect for his private and family life, his home and his correspondence.
2. There shall be no interference by a public authority with the exercise of this right except such as is in accordance with the law and is necessary in a democratic society in the interests of national security, public safety or the economic well-being of the country, for the prevention of disorder or crime, for the protection of health or morals, or for the protection of the rights and freedoms of others.

This is one of the most interesting Articles in the Convention. Because it guarantees the right to respect for private and family life, home and correspondence, it has been interpreted in a variety of ways and for a variety of situations. This Article has been used in many child care cases (*W* v *United Kingdom* (1988) 10 EHRR 29) and by transsexuals seeking recognition about rights of female to male transsexuals being registered as fathers and also seeking recognition about their status (*X, Y and Z* v *United Kingdom* 22 April 1997 and *Rees* v *United Kingdom* (1987) 9 EHRR 56).

There are some limits on the extent to which this right has to be promoted. One of these is that the right does not have to be promoted where there is a need to protect health or morals. The right is watered down by Article 8(2), which allows interference with the right where it is 'necessary in a democratic society' in a number of situations.

In the case of *Guerra* v *Italy* (1998) 26 EHRR 357, the Court found that there had been an infringement of Article 8 and Article 2 where the authorities failed to take practical measures to lower the risk posed by a chemical factory to those who were living one kilometre away. There was a failure to provide essential information about the environment. It may be that nurses who are in contact with gluteraldehyde, for example, would be able to make out a case for infringement of Article 8 where the employer failed to provide the proper information. The Courts have not directly addressed the issue of informed consent in relation to this Article.

Article 8(2) does allow some justification for compulsory treatment. In *Acmanne* v *Belgium* (1983) 40 DR 251 the Court found that compulsory tuberculosis screening was an interference of private life but was justified as necessary to protect health.

Article 9: Freedom of thought, conscience and religion

1. Everyone has the right to freedom of thought, conscience and religion; this right includes freedom to change his religion or belief and freedom, either alone or in community with others and in public or private, to manifest his religion or belief, in worship, teaching, practice and observance.
2. Freedom to manifest one's religion or beliefs shall be subject only to such limitations as are prescribed by law and are necessary in a democratic society in the interests of public safety, for the protection of public order, health or morals, or for the protection of the rights and freedoms of others.

This is an Article in which the protection of freedom of thought, conscience and religion is protected without any qualification. However, the limitations contained in this Article relate to the *manifestations* of these freedoms.

The meaning of what amounts to a belief has had wide interpretation by the Commission, which has held that this includes pacifism. It has been invoked in a case in which a worker who was required to work on Sundays claimed that this infringed his right to observe the sabbath. The Court did not uphold the claim, which some have found surprising (*Stedman* v *United Kingdom* [1997] EHRLR 545).

This Article could be used by those with a specific belief that affects their approach to healthcare. In the case of *Vereniging Rechtswinkels Utrecht* v *The Netherlands* (1986) 46 DR 200, a voluntary association was denied access to a prison after raising concerns about the suicide of a prisoner. The Commission found that aims of an idealistic nature were not within the rights protected by Article 9.

In another health-related case, the Dutch authorities had introduced legislation requiring dairy farmers to become members of the Health Service to prevent tuberculosis among cattle. When the dairy farmers asserted an infringement of Article 9, the Court found that the term 'protection of health' in Article 9(2) could reasonably cover schemes for the prevention of cattle disease (*X* v *The Netherlands* (1962) 5 Yearbook 278).

Article 10: Freedom of expression

1. Everyone has the right to freedom of expression. This right shall include freedom to hold opinions and to receive and impart information and ideas without interference by public authority and regardless of frontiers. This Article shall not prevent states from requiring the licensing of broadcasting, television or cinema enterprises.
2. The exercise of these freedoms, since it carries with it duties and responsibilities, may be subject to such formalities, conditions, restrictions or penalties as are prescribed by law and are necessary in a democratic society, in the interests of national security, territorial integrity or public safety, for the prevention of disorder or crime, for the protection of health or morals, for the protection of the reputation or rights of others, for preventing the disclosure of information received in confidence, or for maintaining the authority and impartiality of the judiciary.

Article 8 can in principle give rise to positive obligations on the state to intervene in relations between private parties. However, the Commission has held that the individual's right to privacy must be weighed against the media's right to freedom of expression under Article 10. The government cannot be criticized under Article 8 for a legal situation where the latter prevailed (*Winer* v *United Kingdom* (1986) 48 D&R 158). Where other remedies exist, such as defamation, that would be sufficient to discharge the government's positive obligations under Article 8.

One of the fascinating aspects of this Article is that it has the real potential to be in conflict with Article 8 and the right to privacy. Article 10 does not allow free speech to be so wide as to include defamation. The rights of others to protect their reputations are covered by one of the restrictions in Article 10(2).

One of the most famous cases on freedom of expression concerned an attempt by the *Sunday Times* to publish an article about the dangers of the anti-morning sickness drug, thalidomide. Because there was already some litigation taking place, the government asked the Court for an injunction to prevent the article being published. The House of Lords granted the injunction and the *Sunday Times* took the case to the European Court of Human Rights, which found that there had been a breach of this Article (*Sunday Times* v *United Kingdom* (1992) 1 EHHR 229).

Article 11: Freedom of assembly and association

1. Everyone has the right to freedom of peaceful assembly and to freedom of association with others, including the right to form and to join trade unions for the protection of his interests.
2. No restrictions shall be placed on the exercise of these rights other than such as are prescribed by law and are necessary in a democratic society in the interests of national security or public safety, for the prevention of disorder or crime, for the protection of health or morals or for the protection of the rights and freedoms of others. This Article shall not prevent the imposition of lawful restrictions on the exercise of these rights by members of the armed forces, of the police or of the administration of the state.

The right to assembly is qualified. It must be *peaceful* assembly and even this right is subject to limitations in the second paragraph. This right is very closely associated with Articles 9 and 10. In the case of *Plattform Arxte für das Leben* v *Austria* (1991) 13 EHRR 204, a group of doctors demonstrating for changes in the abortion laws were disrupted by counter-demonstrations. One of the issues that was considered by the Court was the extent to which the state is required to ensure that conditions exist to allow a peaceful assembly to take place. The Court found that the state had anticipated disruption and had organized a large police presence which showed that their duties under this Article had been considered.

The right to freedom of association should not be confused with the requirements of some professional bodies that membership is a condition of admission to the profession. The Court has held that professional regulatory bodies are not associations within the meaning of Article 11 (*Le Compte, Van Leuvan and De Meyere* v *Belgium* (1982) 4 EHRR 1).

This Article allows people to join associations, and includes the right for everyone to form or join a trade union. There have been a number of cases on this including *National Union of Belgium Police* v *Belgium* (1975) 1 EHRR 578, where the Court found that trade union action was protected. However, the application by workers at GCHQ to overturn a contractual clause that prevented them from joining a trade union was not upheld by the Court (*Council of Civil Service Unions* v *United Kingdom* (1987) 50 DR 228).

Article 12: Right to marry

Men and women of marriageable age have the right to marry and to found a family, according to the national laws governing the exercise of this right.

This Article is not subject to the type of limitations that have been attached to Article 8(2). The limitation in this Article is different and states that the rights and freedoms are subject to domestic law existing in the individual member states. It is not clear why such a restriction should have a place in a European-wide Convention. This means, for example, that the different age limits at which men and women can marry do not need to be similar across all the countries which have signed up to the Convention.

At first sight, this Article appears to be a wide-ranging provision, but the Court has restricted the extent to which this Article can be applied. Where there are already national laws in place regarding marriage the Court will not seek to overturn those. In the case of *Johnston* v *Ireland* (1987) 9 **EHRR** 203, the Court found that the laws in Ireland that prevent divorce, and which also prohibit divorced people from remarrying are lawful. Where countries prohibit marriage by homosexuals or transsexuals, the Court will not overturn such laws either.

This Article will be important in the debate about the recognition of commitment in same sex relationships as well as the right for same sex partners to adopt children. The wording of the Article seems to imply that only married couples can claim the right to found a family. It could be that before a claim can be made about a right to found a family, there must be a demonstration that marriage, according to national law, has taken place. The Article itself talks of 'this right' rather than 'these rights' implying that the two freedoms are co-dependent on each other.

Article 14: Prohibition of discrimination

The enjoyment of the rights and freedoms set forth in this Convention shall be secured without discrimination on any ground such as sex, race, colour, language, religion, political or other opinion, national or social origin, association with a national minority, property, birth or other status.

This Article means that there should be no discrimination on the grounds of sex, race, religion, etc. It is not a right to enjoy lack of discrimination in itself, and can only by used along with another Article which the victim claims has been infringed. This Article means that discrimination is not to be tolerated in connection with enjoyment of the rights in the Convention. There must therefore be a breach of one of the other Articles in the Convention before a further complaint about discrimination can be made.

The established approach to discrimination is that the Court has to ask whether the person has been treated differently because of some objectively irrelevant difference, such as race or sex.

In the case of *Thlimmenos* v *Greece* (6 April 2000) a person who wanted to become an accountant was refused admission to the accountancy regulatory body because he had a conviction for 'insubordination' for refusing to undertake military service which he objected to as a Jehovah's Witness. The Court said that the Convention does not provide free access to any particular profession and discrimination on these grounds is not prohibited. However, his religious convictions meant that his rights had been violated under Article 14 and that he had suffered discrimination. The circumstances of his conviction should have led him to being treated more favourably than others with convictions for subordination. The Court accepted that this amounted to discrimination.

This Article could be used in conjuction with other Articles for a person to complain where there is evidence of 'post code' rationing of services in the UK. This could be used by people who are not receiving healthcare under the NHS but are receiving this through social services for which they are means tested.

Any age discrimination in the health service could be in breach of this Article. This may affect women who want breast screening sooner than the current age limit or others on the waiting lists for an organ donation.

Article 16: Restrictions on political activity of aliens

Nothing in Articles 10, 11 and 14 shall be regarded as preventing the High Contracting Parties from imposing restrictions on the political activity of aliens.

Article 17: Prohibition of abuse of rights

Nothing in this Convention may be interpreted as implying for any state, group or person any right to engage in any activity or perform any act aimed at the destruction of any of the rights and freedoms set forth herein or at their limitation to a greater extent than is provided for in the Convention.

Article 18: Limitation on use of restrictions on rights

The restrictions permitted under this Convention to the said rights and freedoms shall not be applied for any purpose other than those for which they have been prescribed.

Article 16 has the potential to be a restrictive provision and to exclude people classified as aliens from the protections given to those citizens in states that recognize the Convention. The rights of refugees could therefore be restricted under this Article.

Articles 17 and 18 have the potential to limit the rights of the Convention. Many of the applications to the Commission have come from those who are detained, whether in prison or in psychiatric settings, with complaints about infringement of rights and freedoms. However, the wording of Article 18 means that the restrictions which have been built into some of the Articles are express restrictions. The Commission and the Court are limited in the extent to which they can interpret restrictions, particularly for specific groups of persons such as prisoners.

It is not clear why Article 18 has been included in the Convention when there are no similar provisions in the United Nations *Universal Declaration of Human Rights*.

The First Protocol

Article 1: Protection of property

Every natural or legal person is entitled to the peaceful enjoyment of his possessions. No one shall be deprived of his
possessions except in the public interest and subject to the
conditions provided for by law and by the general principles of
international law.

 The preceding provisions shall not, however, in any way
impair the right of a state to enforce such laws as it deems
necessary to control the use of property in accordance with
the general interest or to secure the payment of taxes or
other contributions or penalties.

This Article refers to peaceful enjoyment of possessions rather than a
right of property.

This is the first Article that extends rights to a 'legal person',
which includes companies. What counts as property has been
broadly regarded by the Court and it has already been found to
include patents (*SmithKline and French Laboratories Ltd* v *The Netherlands*
(1990) 66 DR 70). Land and objects have been held to be possessions, as have company shares and goodwill in a business. In health,
there has been a case which ensured that the rights of doctors under
a contract were also upheld (*Association of General Practitioners* v *Denmark*
(1989) 62 DR 226).

However, matters affecting pensions and social security payments
have been more problematic. The Court held in *Müller* v *Austria* (1984)
38 DR 84, that where a fund is created in which a person has an individual share and where a value can be placed on it at any given
moment, it can be regarded as a possession under this Article. Where
the relationship between the contribution and the ultimate benefits
cannot be assessed as precisely, it is unlikely that such a fund would be
considered as a possession (*X* v *United Kingdom* (1970) 13 Yearbook 892).

Article 2: Right to education

No person shall be denied the right to education. In the exercise of any functions which it assumes in relation to education and to teaching, the state shall respect the right of
parents to ensure such education and teaching in conformity
with their own religious and philosophical convictions.

This Article means that the state must have respect for the rights of parents to ensure that teaching is in conformity with their own convictions. This is one of the Articles in which the United Kingdom has chosen to exercise a reservation. This reservation states that the government will only be bound by this Article insofar as it is compatible with the provision of efficient instruction and training and avoidance of unreasonable public expenditure. One famous case on this article was in 1982 where parents challenged the use of corporal punishment in schools on the grounds that this was contrary to their beliefs (*Campbell* v *United Kingdom* (1982) 4 EHRR 293).

The extent to which there should be sex education in schools is a matter that could fall under this Article. The rights of parents are given special scope here and it could be that parents object to the content of sex education in schools. However, the child may want the sex education and the first part of this Article would then apply. The prospect for tension between the pupil, the parent and the school nurse is potentially a problem here.

Article 3: Right to free elections

The High Contracting Parties undertake to hold free elections at reasonable intervals by secret ballot, under conditions which will ensure the free expression of the opinion of the people in the choice of the legislature.

This Article has been included in the Convention to ensure that all countries which have signed up to the provisions of the Convention have a basic form of democracy. This ensures that the citizens of that particular country have the right to vote and to maintain privacy around that vote. The Article also allows the Commission and the Court of Human Rights to deal with claims where a citizen alleges that the elections have not been held at a reasonable interval or where the conditions have interfered with the right to make a free decision.

It is an interesting development that the Protocol moves into the area of democratic expression, and in this way binds the process of the countries in a fundamental manner.

The Sixth Protocol

Article 1: Abolition of the death penalty

The death penalty shall be abolished. No one shall be condemned to such penalty or executed.

Article 2: Death penalty in time of war

A state may make provision in its law for the death penalty in respect of acts committed in time of war or of imminent threat of war; such penalty shall be applied only in the instances laid down in the law and in accordance with its provisions. The state shall communicate to the Secretary General of the Council of Europe the relevant provisions of that law.

These provisions contained in the Convention, which have been incorporated in the Human Rights Act 1998, are largely self-explanatory.

The provisions of these Articles on the death penalty do not supersede or replace one of the exemptions to Article 2, which provides that the legal protection of the right to life can be disregarded where the death penalty has been passed.

Chapter 5
Healthcare and
Human Rights

The right to health

Taken to the extreme the 'right to health' could imply that everyone has a right to a 'guarantee' of perfect health. However, perhaps it would be more realistic to think in terms of the description given by Herman *et al.* (1989: 600) describing it as a 'right to health protection which includes two components, a right to health care and a right to healthy conditions.' At a United Nations workshop in 1979 on the same subject, the Director of the UN Division of Human Rights, Professor Boven, referred to three aspects of health. These have been enshrined in the international instruments on human rights; they are:

1. the declaration of the right to health as a basic human right;
2. the prescription of standards aimed at meeting the health needs of specific groups of persons; and
3. the prescription of ways and means for implementing the right to health.

Health, it could be suggested, may be one of the most important factors in enabling people to lead a dignified life. It has been claimed, however, that rights on their own are of no use for those who lack the basic economic, social and cultural conditions necessary to enjoy them. What is the point of freedom of expression (Article 10) for individuals who cannot express themselves because of a lack of education? What is the point of a right to life (Article 2) for someone who will die due to a lack of medical treatment? In the UK, the system that has been responsible for the provision of healthcare celebrated its fiftieth anniversary in the same year as the enactment of the Human Rights Act 1998. The NHS was born in the same year as the Convention on Human Rights. However, it is apparent that currently the NHS is under enormous scrutiny and criticism. There are problems of financial pressures, finite resources, long waiting lists and lack of access for some to adequate healthcare. The terminology in this field is changing and there is a move towards 'health and social care'. In its 50 years commitment to the Convention the UK has been held by the European Court of Human Rights to have violated the Convention on more than 50 occasions. The UK has been found to have violated almost every Article of the Convention; only Articles 4, 9, and 12 have escaped findings of violations.

Many issues will turn on the distinction between negative rights and positive rights. While negative rights provide protection against interference by others (that is, create duties of non-interference, which are called negative because of their passive nature), positive rights entail active measures from others in order to be fulfilled. The language of the Convention points to an almost exclusive concern with negative rights. There are exceptions, one being Article 2 of the First Protocol dealing with the right to education. In this instance, the UK has claimed the reservation on the extent to which it must act positively.

The provision of health services and health policy

Strategic planning is very important for organizations that are trying to change social conditions. Nearly every issue that affects society, whether it be economic, environmental, developmental, nutritional, health related, cultural or ethnic, will involve a complex set of facets that need to be dealt with. This complexity provides an almost endless supply of challenges. It also supplies 'windows of opportunities' where it would be possible to make a difference, or to effect a change. Strategic planning helps to identify new opportunities. It can also allow the determination of outcomes and may be viewed as a tool of empowerment.

How the provision of public health in the UK may change to meet the demands of the Human Rights Act and a 'rights culture' remains a matter of speculation. By evaluating the current state of healthcare law and medical ethics in the UK it may be possible to make some assessment as to how far those fields already go in upholding human rights, principles and values. Consideration also needs to be given to what extent a rights culture will pose dilemmas for the future development of the disciplines of ethics and health law. Reidy (1999) argued that 'traditionally the "negative" concept of rights has focused on the state not interfering with liberties which could seem to be at odds with a National Health Service in a welfare state. A national health system will involve the state taking steps which clearly intrude on the private lives and beliefs of many individuals.'

Closure of residential homes and relocation of frail and vulnerable residents has been an issue of concern over recent years, particularly where lives may be put at risk. It is possible that Health Authorities may be challenged in the future on the basis of a breach of Article 2 (right to life) when they try to implement plans to close care homes. The Court of Appeal directly applied the rights in Article 8 in 1999 in the case of *R* v *North and East Devon Health Authority ex parte Coughlan* (1999). Pamela Coughlan was a resident in an NHS hospital. The Health Authority wanted to close the hospital and move her to a nursing home. They had made an oral promise to her when she moved into the hospital several years earlier that this would be her 'home for life'. The Court of Appeal found that this proposed move breached her rights under Article 8. It did not matter whether it was reasonable for the Health Authority to consider closure of the hospital; the breach of her rights still occurred. When this case reached the Court of Appeal the dictate of Sir Thomas Bingham was quoted 'The more substantial the interference with human rights, the more the court will require by way of justification before it is satisfied that the decision is reasonable'.

The two primary sections of the Act that affect public authorities are sections 3 and 6, which are aimed at ensuring human rights compliance and directing public authorities. It should be remembered that section 3 of the Human Rights Act is not a concern solely of the courts, but applies to all persons reading legislation. It can therefore be seen to be a potential peg from which the 'human rights' promoting approach to policy can be hung.

Preventative measures under Article 2 include a duty to provide information about known health risks. This approach could have interesting consequences. It is possible that in the future there may be more pressure for the Health Service to take steps to prevent life-threatening conditions. For example, vaccination programmes may need to be widened to cover the 'killer diseases' that appear to be on the increase, such as meningitis and tuberculosis. It is possible that vaccination programmes could be made compulsory. It is foreseeable that individuals could bring an action that aimed to oblige the Health Service to provide vaccination or screening programmes, or alternatively seek compensation for damage which resulted from the lack of such a programme.

As public authorities, NHS bodies need to respect Convention rights in everything they do and this would include the employment of staff. Other bodies, such as GP practices, privatized utilities, nursing agencies, regulatory bodies (for example, the UKCC and GMC) with a mix of both public and private functions, will be constrained by the Act only in regard to their public, not their private, acts.

How the Human Rights Act will relate to healthcare

Fifty years from its inception, the NHS suffers from enormous financial pressures and many patients endure long waiting times. The duty on the Secretary of State for Health for the NHS is: 'the promotion of . . . a comprehensive health service' (NHS Act 1977). Health can be seen as one of the most important factors in enabling an individual to lead a dignified life. The fact that health is referred to in many documents in a human rights context would suggest that health is a social good and not merely a medical, technical or economic problem. However, as medical technology continues to advance at an ever increasing rate, healthcare choices become far more complicated.

The Prime Minister's preface to the government's White Paper on the Act, states that the Act will 'enhance awareness of human rights in our society' (*Rights Brought Home* 1997). By examining the Act and the Convention together it is possible to identify markers that may impact on healthcare policy. There are a number of Convention principles and precedents that can be identified; these can provide some guidance for the provision of healthcare from a human rights perspective. There has been much emphasis on the fact that the Human Rights Act should be seen as 'a living document', which could imply that its interpretation may change with the passage of time and that the precedents previously set by civil law can no longer be relied on (Straw 2000). The Home Secretary, Jack Straw, has indicated that the Act should be seen as an opportunity, not a threat. It safeguards the best British values of fairness, respect for human dignity and inclusiveness. He stressed that he believed 'in time the legislation would help to bring about a culture of rights and responsibilities across the UK. It's about getting all citizens to understand, not just what their rights really are, but also that rights and responsibilities are different sides of the same coin.'

Much of clinical law in the past has focused on the duties expected of clinical staff, rather than focusing on the rights of patients or consumers of the service. Now that the legislation is in force, human rights issues are no longer a matter solely for specialists. Nurses need to become familiar with the sorts of issues that involve infringement of human rights. In the case of complaints, for example, consideration will need to be given to human rights implications when reviewing the nature of the complaint and the way in which it is dealt with. Arguably there are opportunities for nurses to influence social policy, as they may well be the 'experts' whose professional opinion and guidance is sought if cases come before the courts.

The Association of Community Health Councils for England and Wales (ACHCEW) has suggested the Act may prove a useful tool for pursuing a range of issues, which are of concern to patients, and to the way that the NHS operates (Chester 2000). These issues include:

- the inherent unfairness in the NHS complaints procedure;
- clinical negligence cases being inappropriately referred through the complaints procedure;
- mixed sex wards;
- the treatment of older people;
- do not resuscitate orders;
- withdrawal of treatment;
- problems experienced trying to persuade the Health Service Commissioner (Ombudsman) to investigate particular cases;
- long waits in Accident and Emergency departments;
- rationing of expensive treatments;

- closure of care homes;
- access to information relating to public health issues.

It is important to remember that the Convention is primarily concerned with individual rights and freedoms, and not social, political and economic rights. The Convention does not specifically mention rights to a particular quality of health service or the right to social security for example. Inevitably the Act will have different effects for different groups within healthcare:

- the users of the health service,
- those that regulate the service,
- those who are employed within it,
- the service as an employer.

Once people begin to realize the rights that the Convention provides, they are likely to challenge some health service practices. There are a number of Articles which are likely to be of particular importance. Some rights are absolute, for example, the right to life, and the prohibition on torture or inhuman and degrading treatment. Some are qualified, for example, the right to respect for private and family life. Most will be subject to a 'balancing act' with other rights as well as other legitimate interests that the state may have. For example, there are competing interests when considering the right to confidentiality versus the right to free speech. The balance of the public interest must be weighed against the private right.

Activity 3

What are the factors that should be taken into account when weighing up the interests of a community psychiatric nurse who is Hepatitis B positive and the general public? Would these 'interests' change if the nurse were a theatre nurse? Who if anyone should be informed of the nurse's diagnosis?

Discussion points

- How would Article 14 apply?
- Would this need to balance with Article 8?

The users of the health service

NHS bodies are required to answer to the patients they treat. Patients' expectations may stem from standards set out in *The Patient's Charter* but there are fundamental expectations that everything done to patients will be in their interests and done to the highest standards. Increasingly, individuals are going to the courts for a judicial review to ascertain whether 'just' treatment has been received from an NHS body in relation to a decision made, or not made. The NHS patient has had to rely on the laws of negligence and can only sue when harm occurs. *The Patient's Charter* gave no additional legal rights.

It could be argued that patient's rights have been limited even if there are situations where they have been upheld in practice. A new NHS Charter is expected to replace the existing *Patient's Charter* sometime in 2001. This is expected to detail how people can access NHS services, what the NHS commitment is to patients, and the rights and responsibilities patients have within the NHS.

In order for a patient to mount a challenge the individual will need to have a civil right that has been denied him, or interfered with. A claim can only be made on behalf of an individual.

It can be envisaged that issues of resources could prove to be a major concern. Individuals whose life expectancy may be adversely affected by the failure to be provided with that treatment could challenge health authorities that decide not to provide expensive treatments. Beta interferon for those with multiple sclerosis or Taxol for those with breast cancer are two such examples.

Those that regulate the service

The health service, both the NHS and the private sector, has a number of regulators, and all of these regulators will be affected by the provisions of the Act. Within the NHS and the private sector, there are different regulators carrying out similar functions in each of the countries of the United Kingdom. They would, however, all need to be aware of any successful claim made against another regulator to ensure that their own practises were lawful.

In the NHS in England for example, there has already been concern expressed about the decision of the National Institute for Clinical Excellence in England to restrict the use of beta interferon for patients with multiple sclerosis. The basis for reaching this decision, which was that because there was no evidence that everyone benefited, the intention that noone should benefit could be a potential breach of Article 2.

The regulatory bodies that set standards for the NHS and the private sector will be required to consider the provisions of the Human Rights Act when setting standards and giving guidance. For example, where the National Care Standards Commission in England sets standards for the minimum size of rooms that need to be made available before a registration certificate can be provided, this would not appear to be in breach of the Act. However, if the Commission were to say that every care home should only have single rooms, and that no sharing of rooms is permitted, this may be in breach of Article 8. This would be particularly so where a couple wanted to move into a care home for the rest of their lives and wanted to share a room. They may be able to argue that their right to a private life has been interfered with by a standard that means they would have to live apart.

The primary function of the regulatory bodies for the health service is to ensure that there are minimum standards of practice and process in place. Where these conflict with the rights of an individual or a member of staff that are protected under the Act, there is the potential for conflict to occur. In such cases, a patient or a member of staff could make a successful claim that a standard set by one of these regulatory bodies was in breach of the Act. If successful, it is likely that the standard as a whole would have to be changed so that the rights under the Act take precedence over the role of the regulatory body.

Those who are employed within the Health Service

In addition to claims for negligence and breach of contract it is likely that the NHS will have to face claims under the new legislation. If an individual's human rights outlined in the Convention are breached, there can be liability even without negligence.

When considering the NHS as a 'service industry' its staff could be viewed as its most valuable asset. Approximately a million people work for the health service. Their responsibilities focus on elements such as:

- Meeting patients' needs and taking their views into account.
- Respect for confidentiality and patients' dignity and privacy.
- High quality standards.
- The competent provision of wide ranging primary, hospital and preventative services.
- The efficient and effective use of resources.

Employees may be able to contest work schedules which interfere with Article 9 for example; this asserts the right to freedom of religion and by implication the right to observe holy days. Alternatively there may be a case to answer if an employer opens an employee's letter that has been marked 'strictly private and confidential'. In *Campbell* v *United Kingdom* (1992) A 233, the Court found that there was no general right to inspect prisoners' correspondence.

The provisions of Article 8 will apply to nurses where the employer wishes to monitor their phone calls and emails. It is unlawful for a public authority employer to intercept internal communications unless the interference is in accordance with the law and comes within the exception set out in the second paragraph. It might be necessary therefore for an employer to obtain the employee's consent to the monitoring of their telephone calls and emails in advance of any system of surveillance. It might be advisable to obtain individual consent to such surveillance.

Drug testing of nurses and other health staff is a difficult issue, as the requirement for public protection needs to be balanced against possible infringement of Article 8. Where, for example, healthcare staff are taking prescribed medication they are entitled to confidentiality and privacy concerning a medical condition. However, patients in their care are entitled to quality care delivered by practitioners who are safe and not under the influence of any substance that may influence their ability to make reasoned judgements.

The freedom of employees to express their views may conflict with the employer's right to manage the workplace. Employment tribunals will have regard to Article 10 when considering dismissal or discrimination cases based, for example, on failure to follow dress codes. Imposition of dress codes, particularly by a public sector employer, may be deemed an interference of freedom of expression and it is possible that employers may have to justify this expectation.

The service as an employer

Article 8 gives a positive obligation to employers to create conditions where there is respect for private life. In the employment situation it will be relevant whether an aspect of the employee's private life has an effect on their working life or whether working practices have an effect on the employee's private or family life. Where an employer's actions are motivated by an objection to an aspect of the employee's private life, which has no effect on their working life, an Article 8 case is more likely to be successful.

The Public Interest Disclosure Act 1998 has created rights for the 'whistle blower'. Article 10 can also be used by whistle blowers in certain circumstances and strengthens the new whistle blowing legislation. It is possible that employers might try to argue that by accepting a certain type of post an employee accepts certain restrictions on their job. This will not justify interference with the principle of free expression.

Nurses' perspectives and human rights

Nursing shares with other professionals a commitment to the well being of the patient and to a professional practice based on codes of ethics. During the 1980s and 1990s, national and international nurses associations have refined their principles to reflect an increasing commitment to human rights and the protection of the patient.

A number of statements adopted by the International Council of Nurses (ICN 1998; 1999) outline nurses' responsibilities towards human rights. It is noted in *Nurses and Human Rights* that nurses have individual responsibility but they can be more effective if they approach human rights issues as a group. The statement goes on to outline the rights of those in need of care and the rights and duties of nurses.

The ICN is campaigning for nursing organizations to develop strategies which identify the role that individual nurses and other healthcare providers must play to strengthen the links between health and human rights and 'thereby contribute to the prevention of disease and enhance equitable access to healthcare'. It suggests that specifically they need to:

- develop understanding of human rights declarations and instruments;
- create awareness about the vital link between human rights and health and the harmful impact of human rights violations on health;
- provide information to the public about access to health services and how best to use them;
- work with the media, human rights groups, lawyers' associations and policy makers to heighten awareness about the rights approach;
- use specific examples of human rights violations, such as gender

discrimination, female genital mutilation and other forms of violence to demonstrate their harmful consequences on health;
• mainstream human rights and ethics education into all levels of nursing curricula;
• lobby for equity and universal access to comprehensive, cost effective and affordable healthcare and other social services;
• provide information that protects all people from unethical medical experimentation and exposure to harmful procedures and products.

The ICN Position Statement suggests that

> Nurses deal with human rights issues daily, in all aspects of their professional role. Nurses may be pressured to apply their knowledge and skills in ways that are detrimental to patients and others. There is a need for increased vigilance and a requirement to be well informed about how new technology and experimentation can violate human rights. Furthermore nurses are increasingly facing complex human rights issues, arising from conflict situations within jurisdictions, political upheaval and wars. The application of human rights protection should emphasise vulnerable groups such as women, children, elderly, refugees and stigmatised groups

This paragraph is as applicable for nurses in the UK as anywhere else in the world especially in the current climate where nurses are being encouraged both politically and professionally to develop practice and push back the boundaries of care. With the Human Rights Act now in force nurses as part of a 'public authority' must consider their responsibilities in this context.

Some national nurses' associations have also taken initiatives to enshrine human rights principles in their codes of ethics. For example, the Canadian Nurses Association adopted a position statement on human rights in 1991. It endorses the *UN Universal Declaration of Human Rights* and states that 'nurses have an individual and universal responsibility to protect (human rights)' (CNA 1991). The American Nurses Association (ANA 1991) has noted that 'the principle of justice is one point at which issues of ethics and human rights intersect.'

Fundamental ethical obligations identified by ANA for any health care worker include a duty to:

• avoid or minimize harm to patients
• promote individual well-being

- promote the health of vulnerable groups
- promote public health measures
- educate the public on health matters whenever possible.

The ANA (1991) identifies three main responsibilities for nurses:

1. The careful delivery of nursing care in a way that meets the needs of the individual and is consistent with the goals of the individual with respect to level of health and quality of life.
2. Social action and reform to increase the availability of nursing care and to facilitate access to need and healthcare for all.
3. Patient advocacy to ensure that individuals are aware of all options and their consequences and can make informed choices about healthcare.

In the UK, nurses are licenced to practise through the UKCC. The Code of Professional Practice can be regarded as the template against which practice can be measured. While the Code does not specifically refer to 'human rights' it is clear from the way the Code is phrased in its opening statement that the nurses' prime focus of concern is to 'safeguard and promote the interests of individual patients and clients' (UKCC 1992). Now that the Human Rights Act is in force, it is anticipated that the Code will be reviewed.

In addition, it is suggested that nurses must advance and protect their own human rights. This includes the right to be fairly compensated for services rendered, the right to control the quality of practice; the right to engage in 'whistle blowing' when necessary, without reprisals; the right to be able to practise in a safe environment; and the right to be able to engage in independent practice.

With the current moves towards the integration of health and social care there are opportunities for nurses to be hugely influential. It is quite likely that the Courts will look towards the expertise of nurse to articulate best practice and quality care.

When nursing care is viewed as a resource it is crucial that it is distributed fairly and equitably to meet the needs of the population. Achieving fairness and equity is a continuing challenge. As nurses engage in a variety of activities and interventions that have the potential to impinge on the rights of other individuals, the borderline of what is 'usual' or 'normal' practice is increasingly extending into areas of new and 'experimental' practice. As the scope of nursing increases in complexity the professions must become aware of the importance of concerning themselves with the human rights of all individuals who are recipients of nursing care.

It can be argued that the new legislation will encourage professionals to reconsider their responsibilities in the care delivery setting. Particular considerations for nurses could include:

- Does the activity that I am involved in touch on human rights?
- If so, who are the groups who might be affected by the activity?
- Will the impact of any actions taken on those rights be justified in the particular circumstances?

Some of the difficulties in interpreting 'rights' have been distinguishing between moral rights and other rights which are embodied in legislation. Although they may overlap in healthcare, confusion has occurred as to the extent to which 'claiming rights' can be enforced when claiming services. It is anticipated that the Human Rights Act may clarify some of these rights although the extent to which they can be claimed remains a matter of speculation.

While ethical codes and declarations can provide a foundation, education and knowledge are crucial components of any preparation for nurses and healthcare workers if acknowledgement and support of human rights issues are to be effective. Nursing staff clearly have a large amount of contact with patients and must be aware of the issues. Some issues are obvious, for example policies creating age discrimination in treatment and the fact that human dignity demands that patients are no longer left on trolleys in A&E corridors for long periods of time.

Activity 4

A newly appointed ward sister decides to implement a new off-duty rota, so that all staff rotate on to night duty and spend time on day duty, which will make in-service training easier.

Discussion points

- Will there be any breach of Human Rights if the rota is imposed on the staff without any discussion?
- Which Articles will be breached?

Patients' perspectives and human rights

The World Health Report 2000 (WHO 2000) describes patients as users of healthcare services, whether healthy or sick. When an individual becomes ill they do not lose their human rights. An individual who is sick is usually even more vulnerable, even more in need of basic guarantees and assurances. The rights of people in this situation need to be protected and defended.

Patients also have responsibilities. One responsibility is to take care to a large degree of one's own health. Another is to work towards achieving better healthcare and better health systems.

Rights of patients fall into broad groups, which could be classified as:

- Healthcare and humane treatment
- Choice of care
- Acceptable safety
- Adequate information and consent
- Redress of grievances
- Participation and representation
- Health education and healthy environment

Consideration may need to be given to improving access to information about patients' rights. This could be considered to be a crucial element of any strategy to promote patients' rights. The right to privacy contained within Article 8 complements the UK's common law duty of confidentiality. Individuals' rights of access to personal records have been upheld under this Article (*Gaskin* v *UK* [1989] A160).

The Human Rights Act will equip patients and their relatives with the tools and mechanism to identify areas where they are not satisfied with their care and subsequently an increase in complaints may be anticipated. Chester (1998) argues that the NHS complaints procedure does not comply with the requirements of Article 6. The first stage of the procedure may involve consideration of the complaint by the individual being complained about. This leads to questions of independence and impartiality. To some extent this has been recognized in the NHS Plan although there has been no mechanism identified yet to address this.

Article 14 provides for individuals to enjoy Convention rights 'without discrimination on any ground'. This will apply to age discrimination; for example, minimum and maximum age limits for cancer screening. Breaches of this Article cannot be considered in isolation. Article 14 does not operate independently but in conjunction with other Articles. The exclusion of patients over a certain age for organ transplants, for example, could be a breach of Article 2 and, if so, a breach under Article 14 could be considered as well.

Activity 5

How responsive is the NHS complaints procedure to the Human Rights Act?

Discussion points

- Which is the relevant Article?
- Can all complaints be considered?

Children

Although the Convention contains no specific rights for children, it is very significant for family cases. Under paragraph 2 of Article 8, any interference by a public authority, such as taking a child into care, must be in accordance with the law.

The decision by local authorities to make decisions about children in care, without reference to the natural family, has been questioned in the case of *W* v *United Kingdom* [1987] 10 EHRR 29. In that case, a child in voluntary care was placed in foster care by the local authority who then stopped access to his natural parents. The Court found that there had been a breach of Article 8 based on the extent to which the parents had been excluded from the decision made. It did not consider that this exclusion of the parents was 'necessary' within the allowance of the Article.

The Court found that the parents should be involved in the decision making process 'to a degree sufficient to provide them with the requisite protection of their interests' and that this had relevance in the health field as well.

The right to family life may mean that children should not have to languish in care for years on end. In the case of *Barrett* v *Enfield* LBC [1999] 3 WLR 79, the child sued the Local Authority for negligence in failing to arrange his adoption while in their care. Because of the Osman ruling the House of Lords was required to hear the case, even though a similar case five years earlier had been thrown out (*X (Minors)* v *Bedfordshire CC* [1995] AC 633) by the House of

Lords. In the Osman case a ruling was made that immunity for the police for operational reasons was too broad and capable of infringing the human right of protection of life. An absolute rule denying access to courts was disproportionate to the needs of the police.

Activity 6

A 14-year-old girl is brought into the accident and emergency department having been kicked in the stomach at school. The girl tells the nurse she is pregnant but asks her not to tell her mother. The nurse agrees not to tell.

Discussion points

- Which Articles could be considered here?
- Is there any conflict with the rights of the mother?

Confidentiality

Confidentiality and access to records is frequently featured as a concern of patients and nurses alike. Under common law there is no specific right of privacy. Both the General Medical Council (GMC) and the UKCC publish ethical and professional guidance in respect of confidentiality. Article 8, right to respect for private and family life, would cover this issue. While the right of confidentiality in Article 8 is not absolute, the balancing effect of Article 10, the right to exchange opinions and information, may have to be taken into account.

How are victims to be dealt with under this right? In a case dealing with disclosure of medical records (*Z* v *Finland* 25 EHRR 371 (25/2/1997)), a man was convicted of attempted manslaughter after failing to declare his HIV status to a number of sexual partners. At the trial, an order was made that his wife's medical records be disclosed. These records were referred to, along with the wife's identity in the judgment. She went to the European Court of Human Rights and claimed that her rights under Article 8 had been violated. The Court found that it had indeed been necessary for her records to be used in the trial as this was both 'necessary in a democratic society' and proportionate. However the disclosure of her identity was an infringement of her rights and she was awarded compensation. The violation occurred not when the doctor was required to give this evidence, but when the identity of the patient was revealed.

A system such as NHS Direct involves the use of a public telecommunications service to discuss personal matters. Clearly how the service is regulated and controlled to ensure protection of personal information and confidentiality is of utmost importance.

Activity 7

A drug company is interested in collecting data about the prescribing habits of GPs and intends to use the information for commercial gain. The data would be anonymized. The practice nurse is asked to assist in collecting the information.

Discussion points

- Should the consent of the patients involved be obtained?
- Would this practice be in breach of any of the Convention Articles?

Consent

Treatment given without consent is an assault under common law. It is possible that treatment given without consent may amount to inhuman or degrading treatment contrary to Article 3 of the Convention. Experimental medical treatment, which has not been the subject of fully informed consent, could also be in breach of this Article (*X* v *Denmark* 1983 32 DR 282) and may also possibly breach Article 8.

The right to refuse medical treatment can also be supported by Article 9; 'everyone has a right to freedom of thought, conscience and religion . . . to manifest his religion or belief, in worship, teaching, practice and observance'. As in so many other cases, a balancing exercise is required, in order to protect the rights and freedoms of others.

Patients who have made an advance statement about medical treatment should expect to have this respected. Advance statements apply when patients are no longer able to participate in treatment decisions and have become incompetent. The rights of older people may be further protected by the anti-discrimination Article 14, which states that individuals have the same rights regardless of differences in gender, race, culture or age.

Activity 8

A patient on your ward, who has waited nine months for admission, gives her consent for a biopsy. She recovers from the anaesthetic to discover that she has had a mastectomy.

Discussion points

- Which Articles would be concerned with the issue of consent?

Privacy and dignity

The prohibition of torture, inhuman and degrading treatment or punishment is absolute and extends to people subject to any detention, and in general to the manner in which people are treated. These practices could include:

- keeping women prisoners in handcuffs during childbirth,
- general restraint techniques used on patients in order to administer treatment,
- access to proper medical facilities for ill prisoners,
- the dignity of the conditions in which people are maintained,
- the impact of those conditions on their health.

These could all raise challenges on the grounds that they are degrading treatment.

Many healthcare interventions are of an invasive nature and could be defined as degrading; therefore the process of ensuring informed consent from the individual is crucial.

Article 8 protects privacy, family life and home life. The right to privacy has several aspects touching on physical privacy, for example mixed sex wards, the use of surveillance equipment, and personal privacy, for example provision of personal information and issues of sexual orientation.

Activity 9

A patient has been waiting in the A&E department for 24 hours. She has a fractured hip and is waiting for a bed on the orthopaedic ward.

Discussion points

- Which Articles are called into question here?
- Would one right be more persuasive than any other?

Abortion

In the case of *Open Door Counselling Ltd. and Well Woman Clinic Ltd* v *Ireland* (1992) 15 EHRR 244, the Court found that a ban on providing information about abortion was in violation of Article10 even though the practice of abortion is unlawful in Ireland. The Court has also held that there was an infringement of this Article when a person wanting to distribute anti-abortion leaflets before an election was prevented from doing so (*Bowman* v *United Kingdom* (1998) 26 EHRR 1).

Advocates and opponents of abortion and euthanasia may look to the case law of the Convention and the Human Rights legislation for support of their views. To date the European Commission and the Court of Human Rights have preferred to be cautious. There are no clear answers to be found by looking to Strasbourg.

The rights of the healthcare professionals however cannot be ignored. Abortion is a treatment that potentially threatens the integrity of healthcare professionals who believe it to be morally wrong and the Abortion Act 1967 allows 'conscientious objection'. Female genital mutilation, on the other hand, is thought to threaten the integrity of women as a whole and has been made illegal by the Prohibition of Female Circumcision Act 1985.

Transplantation

The exclusion of patients over a particular age from the organ transplant list is likely to breach Article 14. This Article needs to be read in conjunction with the other rights detailed in the Convention. Patients awaiting organ donation may well want to argue that Article 2 is also relevant.

Article 9 protects the rights of those whose beliefs may not accord with mainstream attitudes and probably supports the right of self-determination, for example of Jehovah's witnesses who refuse life-saving treatments in the form of blood transfusions, or other cultures who refuse an organ transplant. In the summer of 2000, Jehovah's Witness elders ruled that accepting blood transfusions will no longer mean excommunication for worshippers, but that they would be seen as 'dissociated' from the faith. It has yet to be seen whether in reality this alters the practice of accepting a blood transfusion, although it may have an impact on parental acceptance on behalf of a child.

Activity 10

A young man urgently needs a kidney transplant and he has been on the waiting list for some time. He has a twin brother who would be an excellent match, but his brother has learning difficulties.

Discussion points

- What are the competing rights to be considered?
- Whose rights should take priority?
- How are these rights to be balanced?

Right to life

There have been occasions when the Courts have recognized that preservation of life might not be a benefit. When caring for the incompetent adult, doctors will be acting lawfully if they withdraw treatment, including hydration and nutrition, providing it is not contrary to the patient's best interests. This is also true of children. Similarly, if competent adults wish treatment to be stopped or withdrawn then the doctor is legally required to accede to the individual's wishes. It has been argued that the position is not so certain in the light of the new legislation. Lord Woolf has commented that 'The principles of law are clearly established, but how you apply those principles to particular facts is often very difficult to anticipate. This may be the current state of English law, but I will argue that the individual rights allowed by the Human Rights Act will, at the very least, significantly curtail – and may even trump – those principles which conflict with them' (*R* v *Portsmouth Hospital NHS Trust* [1999]).

Lord Irvine , the Lord Chancellor, when speaking on the subject said 'Whilst everyone has a right to life, there is not a duty to live (1998).' There will not necessarily be a corresponding duty on others, including doctors, to do everything possible to increase the chances that an endangered life will continue regardless of circumstances. At one extreme there may be an individual who could donate tissue or an organ to save another's life, but is under no obligation to do so. Where the life under threat is that of an individual of full mental capacity, who is determined to end his or her own life, intervention from a third party may amount not to a duty but to an unwarranted interference with the individual's rights.

The cases to date show that this is an issue that is going to have the most extraordinary impact on the provision of health services. In the well publicized case of *R v Cambridgeshire DHA ex parte B* [1995] 1 FLR, 1055 the Court of Appeal overturned the decision of the High Court judge. In that case, Jamie B, who had leukaemia, was seeking an order that Cambridge Health Authority provide innovative treatment. The Court of Appeal said that there was no right to life in law and that the Court had no authority to interfere with the clinical judgement made by the doctors that the treatment would not benefit Jamie. Although there is no guarantee that a similar decision would not be made by the Courts today, it is clear that the provisions of Article 2 would need great consideration.

Right to life issues inevitably reopen questions about abortion practices, euthanasia, withdrawal of treatment, enforced treatment and artificial conception.

Withdrawal of treatment

If common law precedents must give way to the Human Rights Act when withdrawing treatment, the rights threatened might include:

- Right to protection of life under Article 2
- Right not to be subjected to inhuman or degrading treatment under Article 3
- Right to respect for private and family life under Article 8
- Right to protection of individual rights without discrimination under Article 14
- The family's right as 'indirect victims' – not to be subjected to inhuman or degrading treatment under Article 3
- The family's right to respect for family life under Article 8

Activity 11

A patient with a debilitating lung disease, who is ventilated long term, asks for the ventilator alarms to be switched off. He has limited movement but knows how to disconnect his 'tracheostomy' from the ventilator tubing.

Discussion points

- Can someone's competence be called into question if they are on long-term ventilation?
- Which Articles are relevant?

Treatment choices

It is highly likely that following implementation of the Act that patients will start demanding the right to life-saving treatment by relying on Article 2, which states that 'Everyone's right to life shall be protected by law'.

In the past it has been possible to withdraw or withhold treatment if thought to be futile and of no benefit to the patient. It is possible that this may be more the subject of a challenge of a breach of Article 2.

Determining patient need has varied widely throughout the country and led to what has been called 'postcode rationing'. If publicly funded treatments are available in one area, others may have difficulty defending a decision made which refuses treatment in that area. Patients suffering from multiple sclerosis or Alzheimer's Disease may request drugs that are not universally available and expensive. This may infringe Article 2.

It is unclear under Article 8 whether this right means that all infertile couples are entitled to treatment. It is possible that individuals might try to rely on Article 12, which is concerned with the right to marry and found a family, in order to obtain fertility treatment, such as IVF, or even Viagra.

Non-consensual treatment on the other hand may result in a claim of inhuman or degrading treatment, thus breaching Article 3. Patients who have made an advance statement about medical treatment should expect to have this respected.

Disregarding patient's wishes may result in a claim under Article 8. Similarly as in the case of Coughlan (see below), a resident of a nursing home could seek redress if asked to move because of its closure due to lack of funds. Here there would be a failure to show respect for the patient's life in that home.

Resources

It is possible that the assertion of lack of resources may not continue to provide the health services with a defence for breaching Convention rights. The judges are going to have to balance the right to life of the individual against the clinical judgements of doctors and nurses about the risks and benefits of the proposed treatment. This will not be an easy matter. It is less clear how the judges are going to balance the right to life over the decision of the Health Authority about how it is to spend its resources over a year.

However, this 'postcode lottery' of healthcare provision could be seen as a denial of persons' rights. When treatment available in one area is not available in another it can be argued that this is inequitable and that similar treatments should be available in all areas.

In this respect Article 8 has already been used to prevent the closure of a hospital in Exeter where a patient had been promised a home for life (*R v North and East Devon Health Authority ex parte Coughlan* (1999)). The Court of Appeal maintained that it did not matter that it was reasonable for the Health Authority to consider closing the hospital, there had been a breach of human rights.

If the Act had been in place at the time of the case of Child B, who had leukaemia and was refused treatment by Cambridge Health Authority, it is possible that the courts may have made a different decision. The child's parents requested that the health authority pay for the child to have further chemotherapy and a bone marrow transplant in a private hospital. The health authority's refusal was upheld by the Court of Appeal. Under Article 2 an argument could be made that the state did not fulfil its duty to safeguard life.

Operations that are cancelled and delayed resulting in the death of a patient may be interpreted as a failure to give treatment when the patient's life can be saved, and result in a violation of Article 2. Whilst it is not unlawful to withhold futile treatment under the Act, actively withdrawing treatment based on quality of life is more difficult.

Article 14 may give added protection to the rights of older people under the Act where decisions are made to withhold treatment based on an upper age, for example when some surgery, renal dialysis or transplantation is required. This Article states that everyone has the same rights under the Convention, regardless of differences of religion, sex, race, colour, language or age.

Couples wishing to undergo fertility treatment, which often attracts very limited funding under the NHS, may make a challenge under Article 12 (the right to marry and found a family). It may be that only married couples could take action under Article 12.

Mental health and learning disabilities

In health terms, it is possible to see that Article 3 is a right that might be used more in the fields of mental health and learning difficulties than in some other areas. The case law from the European Court of Human Rights suggests some ambivalence about the application of this right in all settings. In *Tomasi* v *France* (1993) 15 **EHRR** 1, the Court made a ruling that the right was breached where the applicant suffered physical assault, withdrawal of food and a range of other deprivations. In the same year, however, the Court found in the case of *Herczegfalvy* v *Austria* (1993) 15 **EHRR** 437 that the applicant did not suffer a breach of his rights under this article when he was force-fed and given drugs while on hunger strike. He was also handcuffed to his bed for a period of weeks. Mr Tomasi was not detained in a mental health setting but Mr Herczegfalvy was detained as a 'mentally deranged offender'. The Court found that there was no breach of Article 3 as:

> medical authorities can decide, on the basis of the recognized rules of medical science, on the therapeutic methods to be used, if necessary by force, to preserve the physical and mental health of patients who are entirely incapable of deciding for themselves and for whom they are therefore responsible . . . the established principles of medicine are admittedly in principle decisive in these cases; as a genuine rule, a measure which is a therapeutic necessity cannot be regarded as inhuman or degrading. The court must nevertheless satisfy itself that the medical necessity has been convincingly shown to exist.
>
> It does not seem therefore that it is necessary for the force feeding to be given only where the person is suffering from a mental illness.

In *Winterwerp* v *the Netherlands* (1979) 2 **EHRR** 387, the Court looked at the definition of 'persons of unsound mind' and said that this term could not be given a definite meaning especially as the attitude of society changes towards those with mental illness. Any definite meaning would also trap the countries where advances in treatment were being decided. What the Court did say was that a person would not be regarded as being of unsound mind 'simply because his views or behaviour deviate from the norms prevailing in a particular society'.

The test for detention set out in the Winterwerp case is that:

- 'objective medical expertise' must show that a person is of unsound mind
- this test does not apply in emergency cases
- the mental disorder must be of a kind 'warranting compulsory confinement'
- continuing detention is justified only where the disorder persists
- detention must be in accordance with national law

It must be remembered that any detention must be sanctioned by and comply with UK laws, for example under the Mental Health Act 1983. This law is currently under review to ensure that its provisions do not breach Convention requirements.

The Commission is likely to find that treatment for those in detention is a requirement for the authorities. In *Hurtado* v *Switzerland I* (1997) 24 EHRR 423, there was an obligation to provide medical treatment for a prisoner who had not been given treatment for his broken ribs after eight days in detention. There was a duty to safeguard the welfare of those in detention.

Chapter 6
Activities and
Commentary

Introduction

This section aims to develop the activities that have been posed throughout the text of the previous chapters. How the Act will work in practice is uncertain and remains speculative. It has been suggested that the potential for reinterpretation of the existing legislation is vast and that the Act has major implications for those working in public authorities. Chapter 4 examines the Articles in detail. The activities are based on case histories that consider issues which have proved to be of concern to patients and nurses, and relate them to the corresponding Articles in order to demonstrate how the Act might be applied in practice.

Activity 1: Changes in healthcare

Think of one aspect of health that has changed over the past 100 years.

Discussion points

- What were the values that were associated with it at that time?
- What are the values that are now associated with this change?

Commentary

The National Health Service celebrated its fiftieth anniversary in the year that the Human Rights Act received royal assent. Several texts analysing the health service have subsequently been published describing its progress. The NHS Act 1977 established a 'comprehensive health service to secure the improvement in the physical and mental health of the people . . . and the prevention, diagnosis and treatment of illness.' What it did not do was establish an individual entitlement for treatment of particular illnesses. It is only since the 1990s that there has been greater recognition given to patients' interest and rights. The publication of documents such as the *Citizen's Charter* and the *Patient's Charter* has had an effect on raising the expectations of users of the NHS.

It has been argued that the healthcare attempts to serve the interests of both the individual and the community result in unavoidable tensions. As individuals or 'consumers' we have an expectation that the health services will be characterized by trust, confidentiality and a willingness to meet the need for care in a way that ensures the best possible outcome. Community expectations, however, centre on equitable distribution of services, responsiveness to local views, effective disease prevention and health promotion. It is inevitable that however the health service is organized, these diverse interests will come into conflict. The attempt to balance the interests of citizens and users will lie at the heart of many of the most fiercely debated issues in healthcare policy.

Activity 2: Code of Conduct

Look at the UKCC Code of Conduct.

Discussion point

• Do you think there are any principles that could be added to the Code which specifically deal with human rights?

Commentary

The United Kingdom Central Council for Nursing, Midwifery and Health Visiting (UKCC) is the regulatory body for the nursing, midwifery and health visiting professions and was established in November 1980. The organization, along with the four National Boards, was set up by statute and replaced the pre-existing statutory and training bodies. The UKCC is entirely funded by registrants' fees. Its key tasks are to: maintain a register of qualified nurses, midwives and health visitors; set standards for nursing, midwifery and health visiting education, practice and conduct; provide advice for nurses, midwives and health visitors on professional standards; and consider allegations of misconduct or unfitness to practise due to ill health.

At a meeting of the UKCC in June 2000, President Alison
Norman stated:

> Protecting the public from practitioners who are alleged to be unsafe to
> practise is at the very heart of what we are here to do. In order to be effective
> in this work and to continue to enjoy the confidence of the public and the
> professions alike justice must be seen to be done in all our professional
> conduct work. The Human Rights Act has focused our attention on the
> need to explain these decisions more systematically, but we are going further
> than is laid down in the Act.'

Activity 3: Whose interests?

What are the factors that should be taken into account when weighing up the interests of a community psychiatric nurse who is
Hepatitis B positive and the general public? Would these 'interests'
change if the nurse were a theatre nurse? Who if anyone should be
informed of the nurse's diagnosis?

Discussion points

- How would Article 14 apply?
- Would this need to balance with Article 8?

Commentary

The Convention does not guarantee freedom from discrimination by
itself. A claim under Article 14 must be attached to a claim arising
from one of the other substantive rights of the Convention. This
Article reinforces the ethical principle that an individual should
refrain from discriminating against another individual.

Article 8 covers a wide range of issues, including the right to
confidentiality. This right does not have to be promoted where
there is a need to protect 'health or morals'. In X v Y [1988] 2 All
ER 649, the exercise in balancing the public interests led to a
court order forbidding the disclosure of confidential information.
In that case, employees of a Health Authority supplied a newspa-
per with the names of two doctors with AIDS, who were still
practising medicine. The judge concluded that the public interest
in maintaining confidence in the circumstances of AIDS was a
significant and fundamental one. The expert testimony which he
accepted suggested that preventing the spread of the virus would

be seriously impeded if those who thought that they might have been infected could not disclose this fact to health professionals in the knowledge that the information would remain confidential. The public interest in the freedom of the press was outweighed in this respect.

If healthcare professionals become infected with HIV or Hepatitis, there are several publications that can be referred to in respect of their professional responsibilities. These include: the UKCC Registrar's letter and statement (dated 6 April 1993); GMC's booklet *HIV and AIDS: the ethical considerations* (October 1995); and the guidance of the Expert Advisory Group on AIDS (March 1994), *AIDS/HIV – Infected Health Care Workers: Guidance on the Management of Infected Health Care Workers.*

Activity 4: Employment rotas

A newly appointed ward sister decides to implement a new off-duty rota, so that all staff rotate on to night duty and spend time on day duty, which will make in-service training easier.

Discussion points

- Will there be any breach of Human Rights if the rota is imposed on the staff without any discussion?
- Which Articles will be breached?

Commentary

Under Article 8 there may be a breach as the 'working arrangements' may be detrimental to family life. This Article protects privacy, family life and home life from unwarranted intrusion by public authorities. It also requires that positive action be taken in some circumstances to promote respect for such privacy. Article 8 gives a positive obligation to employers to create conditions where there is respect for private life.

The Human Rights Act will not create direct rights for employees whose employers are not public authorities. However, the Act will have relevance to all employment claims because courts and tribunals are included within the definition of 'public authorities' within the Human Rights Act and thus will have an obligation to comply with the Convention when deciding cases. All employment tribunal cases therefore will come within Article 6

Article 11 gives the right to be represented by a trade union. The Employment Relations Act 1999 has made significant improvements to employment conditions, including the right for workers to be accompanied by a trade union official in disciplinary and grievance hearings.

Activity 5: Complaints

How responsive is the NHS complaints procedure to the Human Rights Act?

Discussion points

- Which is the relevant Article?
- Can all complaints be considered?

Commentary

Article 6 would be pertinent here. In determination of civil rights and obligations, everyone is entitled to a fair and public hearing, within a reasonable time, by an independent and impartial tribunal, established by law. However, for Article 6 to be relevant, the matter under consideration must be a civil right. For example, failure to treat or negligent care would be accepted as complaints about civil rights, but a complaint about rudeness would not. Judgments should be made publicly except where the publicity would prejudice the interests of justice.

Article 6 applies to both criminal and civil tribunals, including inquests. The requirement for fair and public hearings may prove problematic for the NHS complaints procedure where the mechanism for handling patients' concerns may not comply with the requirements of the Act. Review panels may not be independent and there is no right of appeal to a higher court. Inquests too may come under scrutiny. The requirement that proceedings be heard in public may prove useful when seeking to ensure that the findings of private inquiries are made public.

The NHS complaints system was the subject of major review and reconstruction in 1994 when the Wilson Report *Being Heard* was published. The report highlighted the complexity of the system that existed at that time, which was experienced by complainants, such as lack of information about complaints, delays and problems in obtaining a satisfactory response. Following consultation the procedure was reviewed and guidance issued in 1996. The new system was intended to be more responsive and open.

Activity 6: Children

A 14-year-old girl is brought into the accident and emergency department having been kicked in the stomach at school. The girl tells the nurse she is pregnant but asks her not to tell her mother. The nurse agrees not to tell.

Discussion points

- Which Articles could be considered here?
- Is there any conflict with the rights of the mother?

Commentary

There have been cases through the Courts that have been based on making an assessment of the 'best interests of the child'. This approach reflects the importance placed on the welfare of the child as outlined in the Children Act 1989.

There may be competing interests of the child and the parent. Articles to be considered include Article 8 as the child has a right to privacy and confidentiality. However, there have been cases that have recognized the rights of parents to be involved in decisions relating to the care of children under the 'right to family life' aspect of Article 8.

It is possible for children to be involved in treatment decisions and give consent for treatment. A competent child might look to Article 5 (which protects the right to liberty and security), Article 8 (privacy and security) and Article 14 (prohibition of discrimination) when asserting the right to be in control of treatment choices.

Activity 7: Confidentiality and research

A drug company is interested in collecting data about the prescribing habits of GPs and intends to use the information for commercial gain. The data would be anonymized. The practice nurse is asked to assist in collecting the information.

Discussion points

- Should the consent of the patients involved be obtained?
- Would this practice be in breach of any of the Articles?

Commentary

A breach of confidentiality is likely to be a breach of the UK's obligation under Article 8(1) to preserve the right to respect for private life. However, Article 8(2) provides certain exceptions to that right, for example for the prevention of crime and disorder, the protection of health and the protection of the rights and freedoms of others.

There has been concern that confidential information held in patients' records has been made freely available to too many people in the course of research and information gathering. This has been the subject of a judicial review in *R* v *Department of Health, ex parte Source Informatics* (2000). In this case there was an application for declaratory relief by a data collection company on the grounds that the Department of Health's policy of discouraging GPs and pharmacists from disclosing prescription or dispensing information was erroneous in law. The Court was in favour of maintaining patients' confidentiality. It declared that it was unlawful to release confidential information to commercial concerns for research purposes without the consent of the particular patients concerned, even if the information was anonymized. The Department of Health advice was correct and did not breach Article 10.

Activity 8: Consent to treatment

A patient on your ward, who has waited nine months for admission, gives her consent for a biopsy. She recovers from the anaesthetic to discover that she has had a mastectomy.

Discussion point

- Which Articles would be concerned with the issue of consent?

Commentary

Consent is a fundamental issue under the Human Rights Act.

It is now an established part of law that no treatment may be given to an individual, whether it be clinical or nursing, unless the patient has consented to the treatment. If health professionals proceed with treatment without the patient's consent, they are vulnerable to an action in battery.

Consent is the legal means by which the patient gives a valid authorization for treatment or care. The legal basis of consent is therefore identical to the professional requirement that nurses need consent before carrying out any treatment. The case law on consent has established three requirements that must all be satisfied before any consent given by a patient can be sufficient:

1. The consent should be given by someone with the mental ability to do so.
2. Sufficient information should be given to the patient.
3. The consent must be freely given.

Coercion or manipulation of the patient would tend to imply that consent has not been obtained voluntarily. In this situation, even where the patient signs a consent form, the consent will have been obtained in an unlawful manner and the consent will not be valid.

In this context, a consent form is important evidence although it should never be the only factor taken into account in establishing that full and proper consent has been obtained.

Under the Human Rights Act, it is possible that the patient could assert that there has been a breach of Article 3 and Article 10. Under Article 3, the patient may argue that she has been subject to degrading treatment in that she has suffered a mastectomy where she did not give her permission for this to occur. Under Article 10, the patient would be able to show that her right to freedom of expression includes the right to receive information. Although there is a provision in Article 10 that allows a restriction on this right where it is for the protection of health or morals, it is difficult to see how a surgeon could rely on this defence in the case of an individual patient.

Activity 9: Waiting for a bed

A patient has been waiting in the A&E department for 24 hours. She has a fractured hip and is waiting for a bed on the orthopaedic ward.

Discussion points

- Which rights are called into question here?
- Would one right be more persuasive than any other?

Commentary

Here the right to be free from 'inhuman and degrading treatment', Article 3, would apply. Depending on the level of information made available, Article 10 may also be called into question. As with many of the other articles, Article 8 may also have been breached.

Lack of proper care for patients with a serious illness or following an accident could violate Article 3. Over the past few years many organizations, including the RCN, have highlighted what has become known as the 'winter pressures' where patients lie in crowded corridors or overcrowded cubicles waiting to be transferred to a bed on a ward or specialist area. They are often left exposed with very little privacy and dignity. They may also be left untreated, in pain and without medication for many hours, this could amount to a breach of Article 3. The government has invested a significant sum of money to try to tackle the problem which is being addressed in a number of ways.

It is possible that the continued use of mixed sex accommodation may also bring a challenge under Article 3. Many hospitals have failed to abolish all mixed sex accommodation despite a government commitment. This type of accommodation has lead to patients being treated in an undignified manner with a lack of privacy. Lack of resources are unlikely to be suitable defence for NHS bodies who may be challenged.

Activity 10: Organ donation

A young man urgently needs a kidney transplant and he has been on the waiting list for some time. He has a twin brother who would be an excellent match, but his brother has learning difficulties.

Discussion points

- What are the competing rights to be considered?
- Whose rights should take priority?
- How are these rights to be balanced?

Commentary

There are three main competing rights to consider in this scenario:

- The states obligation to preserve life
- The right to be free from a degrading and inhuman condition
- The right to self-determination and self-expression.

The Convention of Human Rights makes no specific reference to transplantation. Transplants from live donors can be undertaken for the therapeutic benefit of the recipient and where there is no suitable organ available from a deceased person and no other alternative therapeutic method of comparable effectiveness. In this case though, it would be difficult to obtain the necessary consent from someone with learning difficulties, and therefore difficult to establish that the organ was being donated willingly and for entirely altruistic purposes. Within the UK the Unrelated Live Transplant Regulation Authority (ULTRA) also governs live organ donation. The purpose of ULTRA is to prevent the sale of organs for transplantation and to ensure that any organ donation is entirely altruistic. Any coercion or persuasion could amount to a breach of the donor's rights, Article 3 for example. There is also an obligation to warn the individual of any health risks associated with the surgery.

This is an area where some doctors and nurses exercise conscientious objection, as performing surgery on a healthy donor for the benefit of a third party is not of a direct therapeutic purpose to the donor and will carry an element of risk.

Activity 11: Treatment choices

A patient, with a debilitating lung disease, who is ventilated long term asks for the ventilator alarms to be switched off. He has limited movement but knows how to disconnect his 'tracheostomy' from the ventilator tubing.

Discussion points

- Can someone's competence be called into question if they are on long-term ventilation?
- Which Articles are relevant?

Commentary

Consideration needs to be given to Article 2. Allowing a person to die by withholding treatment is permissible, although active actions to hasten death are not. An adult who has 'capacity' and is deemed competent has autonomy to decide not to have further treatment even if the outcome is that he will die. Common law has established the legally binding nature of clear and competent advance statements about treatment that address particular circumstances, which may arise later when a person is no longer able to make their own decisions.

In this case, the first decision would have to be whether the patient was competent to make his own treatment decision. If so, then it is appropriate to consider why he wants the alarms switched off rather than have the whole machine switched off. If it is because he wants to choose his own moment to disconnect the tubing, it may be that his rights under Article 3 need to be considered. If he considers that making his own decision to disconnect himself from the equipment is appropriate for him, he may be able to argue that to have another person do this for him would amount to degrading treatment. However, the hospital may argue that they have to retain control over such a piece of equipment and that they need to be aware of the decision that is being made by the patient and to be an integral part of that process. In this case, the hospital may feel that if the patient raised a claim under Article 10, this freedom of expression about how he was choosing to die was subject to the limitation that this was not permissible in overall health terms.

Conclusion

When the UN *Universal Declaration of Human Rights* was first agreed it established the principle that human rights are indivisable and universal. Incorporation of the European Convention into UK law is long overdue especially if the UK is to remain credible when playing a key role in the defence of human rights internationally.

People have rights simply because they are human – they have the right to lead a dignified and human life. It would appear to be impossible for a legal system to consistently claim to respect human rights without acknowledging a positive right to healthcare. The introduction of the new legislation, which incorporates the European Convention on Human Rights into British law, could result in profound effects on the provision of healthcare throughout the UK.

Often when things go wrong, many patients and relatives are more concerned with being given an explanation or information and possibly an apology. Rarely is the intention to seek damages but recognition that something went wrong and a wish to prevent the same thing occurring to someone else.

When the Home Secretary introduced the Human Rights Bill into the House of Commons, he commented that: 'Those freedoms alone are not enough; they need to be complemented by positive rights that individuals can assert when they believe that they have been treated unfairly by the state, or that the state and its institutions have failed properly to protect them.'

Chapter 7
Resources

Understanding case references

The cases that have been heard at the European Court of Human Rights are given a reference number. This allows anyone to search the text of the case. For example:

Trivedi v *United Kingdom* (1997) EHRLR 521

The applicant was a person called Trivedi who made a claim that a violation had occurred by the United Kingdom. The full text can be found in the European Human Rights Law Reports (EHRLR) for the year 1997 at page 521.

The law reports can be found at main university libraries and at the Law Society library in Chancery Lane, London, WC2

Useful websites

Sources of Convention law can be found on the following websites:
- Court of Human Rights: http://www.dhcour.coe.fr
- Commission: http://www.dhcommhr.coe.fr
- Human Rights Unit – Home Office:
  http://www.homeoffice.gov.uk
- International Council of Nurses:
  http://www.icn.ch/pshumrights.htm

Useful addresses

Human Rights Information Centre
Human Rights Information Centre
Council of Europe
67075 STRASBOURG CEDEX
France
Tel: (33) 88 41 20 24
Fax: (33) 88 41 27 04

The following may be obtained from the Human Rights
Information Centre:

* the text of the Convention,
* information regarding reservations and derogations,
* general information about the Convention system.

United Nations Centre for Human Rights
United Nations Office at Geneva
8–14 Avenue de la Paix
1211 Geneva 10, Switzerland
Tel: (41) 22 917 3924
Fax: (41) 22 917 0213

United Nations Conventions

* Convention on the Prevention and Punishment of the Crime of Genocide (entered into force in 1951)
* International Convention on the Elimination of All Forms of Racial Discrimination (entered into force in 1969)
* Convention on the Elimination of All Forms of Discrimination against Women (entered into force in 1981)
* Convention against Torture and Other Cruel, Inhuman or Degrading Treatment or Punishment (entered into force in 1987)
* Convention on the Rights of the Child (entered into force in 1990)
* International Convention on the Protection of the Rights of All Migrant Workers and Members of their Families (adopted in 1990, not yet in force)

Books on human rights

Judicial Review and the Human Rights Act, Gordon and Ward, Cavendish Publishing Ltd, 2000

The Strasbourg Caselaw, Gordon and Ward, Sweet and Maxwell, 2000

Health and Human Rights; a reader, Mann, Gruskin et al, Routledge, 1999

Human Rights in the Health Service, Marion Chester, Association of Community Health Councils for England and Wales, 1999

Medical Law, Kennedy and Grubb, 2nd edn, Butterworths, 1994, has a powerful section dealing with extracts from the Nuremberg trials and the impact this has had on trials in medical research.

Appendix 1
The Human Rights Act 1998

ARRANGEMENT OF SECTIONS

Introduction

Section
1.   The Convention Rights.
2.   Interpretation of Convention rights.

Legislation
3.   Interpretation of legislation.
4.   Declaration of incompatibility.
5.   Right of Crown to intervene.

Public authorities
6.   Acts of public authorities.
7.   Proceedings.
8.   Judicial remedies.
9.   Judicial acts.

Remedial action
10.   Power to take remedial action.

Other rights and proceedings
11.   Safeguard for existing human rights.
12.   Freedom of expression.
13.   Freedom of thought, conscience and religion.

Derogations and reservations
14.   Derogations.
15.   Reservations.
16.   Period for which designated derogations have effect.
17.   Periodic review of designated reservations.

Judges of the European Court of Human Rights
18.   Appointment to European Court of Human Rights.

Parliamentary procedure
19.   Statements of compatibility.

Supplemental
20.   Orders etc. under this Act.
21.   Interpretation, etc.
22.   Short title, commencement, application and extent.

SCHEDULES

<table>
<tr><td>Schedule 1</td><td>-</td><td>The Articles.</td></tr>
<tr><td>Part I</td><td>-</td><td>The Convention.</td></tr>
<tr><td>Part II</td><td>-</td><td>The First Protocol.</td></tr>
<tr><td>Part III</td><td>-</td><td>The Sixth Protocol.</td></tr>
<tr><td>Schedule 2</td><td>-</td><td>Remedial Orders.</td></tr>
<tr><td>Schedule 3</td><td>-</td><td>Derogation and Reservation.</td></tr>
<tr><td>Part I</td><td>-</td><td>Derogation.</td></tr>
<tr><td>Part II</td><td>-</td><td>Reservation.</td></tr>
<tr><td>Schedule 4</td><td>-</td><td>Judicial Pensions.</td></tr>
</table>

An Act to give further effect to rights and freedoms guaranteed under the European Convention on Human Rights; to make provision with respect to holders of certain judicial offices who become judges of the European Court of Human Rights; and for connected purposes.
[9th November 1998]

BE IT ENACTED by the Queen's most Excellent Majesty, by and with the advice and consent of the Lords Spiritual and Temporal, and Commons, in this present Parliament assembled, and by the authority of the same, as follows:-

Introduction
The Convention Rights.

1. - (1) In this Act "the Convention rights" means the rights and fundamental freedoms set out in-

(a) Articles 2 to 12 and 14 of the Convention,
(b) Articles 1 to 3 of the First Protocol, and
(c) Articles 1 and 2 of the Sixth Protocol,
     as read with Articles 16 to 18 of the Convention.

(2) Those Articles are to have effect for the purposes of this Act subject to any designated derogation or reservation (as to which see sections 14 and 15).

(3) The Articles are set out in Schedule 1.

(4) The Secretary of State may by order make such amendments to this Act as he considers appropriate to reflect the effect, in relation to the United Kingdom, of a protocol.

(5) In subsection (4) "protocol" means a protocol to the Convention-

(a) which the United Kingdom has ratified; or
(b) which the United Kingdom has signed with a view to ratification.

(6) No amendment may be made by an order under subsection (4) so as to come into force before the protocol concerned is in force in relation to the United Kingdom.

Interpretation of Convention rights.

2. - (1) A court or tribunal determining a question which has arisen in connection with a Convention right must take into account any-

(a) judgment, decision, declaration or advisory opinion of the European Court of Human Rights,

(b) opinion of the Commission given in a report adopted under Article 31 of the Convention,

(c) decision of the Commission in connection with Article 26 or 27(2) of the Convention, or

(d) decision of the Committee of Ministers taken under Article 46 of the Convention,
whenever made or given, so far as, in the opinion of the court or tribunal, it is relevant to the proceedings in which that question has arisen.

(2) Evidence of any judgment, decision, declaration or opinion of which account may have to be taken under this section is to be given in proceedings before any court or tribunal in such manner as may be provided by rules.

(3) In this section "rules" means rules of court or, in the case of proceedings before a tribunal, rules made for the purposes of this section-

(a) by the Lord Chancellor or the Secretary of State, in relation to any proceedings outside Scotland;

(b) by the Secretary of State, in relation to proceedings in Scotland; or

(c) by a Northern Ireland department, in relation to proceedings before a tribunal in Northern Ireland-

(i) which deals with transferred matters; and

(ii) for which no rules made under paragraph (a) are in force.

Legislation

Interpretation of legislation.

3. - (1) So far as it is possible to do so, primary legislation and subordinate legislation must be read and given effect in a way which is compatible with the Convention rights.

(2) This section-

(a) applies to primary legislation and subordinate legislation whenever enacted;
(b) does not affect the validity, continuing operation or enforcement of any incompatible primary legislation; and
(c) does not affect the validity, continuing operation or enforcement of any incompatible subordinate legislation if (disregarding any possibility of revocation) primary legislation prevents removal of the incompatibility.

Declaration of incompatibility.

4. - (1) Subsection (2) applies in any proceedings in which a court determines whether a provision of primary legislation is compatible with a Convention right.

(2) If the court is satisfied that the provision is incompatible with a Convention right, it may make a declaration of that incompatibility.

(3) Subsection (4) applies in any proceedings in which a court determines whether a provision of subordinate legislation, made in the exercise of a power conferred by primary legislation, is compatible with a Convention right.

(4) If the court is satisfied-

(a) that the provision is incompatible with a Convention right, and
(b) that (disregarding any possibility of revocation) the primary legislation concerned prevents removal of the incompatibility, it may make a declaration of that incompatibility.

(5) In this section "court" means-

(a) the House of Lords;
(b) the Judicial Committee of the Privy Council;
(c) the Courts-Martial Appeal Court;
(d) in Scotland, the High Court of Justiciary sitting otherwise than as a trial court or the Court of Session;
(e) in England and Wales or Northern Ireland, the High Court or the Court of Appeal.

(6) A declaration under this section ("a declaration of incompatibility")-

(a) does not affect the validity, continuing operation or enforcement of the provision in respect of which it is given; and
(b) is not binding on the parties to the proceedings in which it is made.

Right of Crown to intervene.

5. - (1) Where a court is considering whether to make a declaration of incompatibility, the Crown is entitled to notice in accordance with rules of court.

(2) In any case to which subsection (1) applies-

(a) a Minister of the Crown (or a person nominated by him),
(b) a member of the Scottish Executive,
(c) a Northern Ireland Minister,
(d) a Northern Ireland department,

is entitled, on giving notice in accordance with rules of court, to be joined as a party to the proceedings.

(3) Notice under subsection (2) may be given at any time during the proceedings.

(4) A person who has been made a party to criminal proceedings (other than in Scotland) as the result of a notice under subsection (2) may, with leave, appeal to the House of Lords against any declaration of incompatibility made in the proceedings.

(5) In subsection (4)-

"criminal proceedings" includes all proceedings before the Courts-Martial Appeal Court; and "leave" means leave granted by the court making the declaration of incompatibility or by the House of Lords.

Public authorities
Acts of public authorities.

6. - (1) It is unlawful for a public authority to act in a way which is incompatible with a Convention right.

(2) Subsection (1) does not apply to an act if-

(a) as the result of one or more provisions of primary legislation, the authority could not have acted differently; or
(b) in the case of one or more provisions of, or made under, primary legislation which cannot be read or given effect in a way which is compatible with the Convention rights, the authority was acting so as to give effect to or enforce those provisions.
(3) In this section "public authority" includes-

(a) a court or tribunal, and
(b) any person certain of whose functions are functions of a public nature,
but does not include either House of Parliament

or a person exercising functions in connection with proceedings in Parliament.

(4) In subsection (3) "Parliament" does not include the House of Lords in its judicial capacity.

(5) In relation to a particular act, a person is not a public authority by virtue only of subsection (3)(b) if the nature of the act is private.

(6) "An act" includes a failure to act but does not include a failure to-

(a) introduce in, or lay before, Parliament a proposal for legislation; or
(b) make any primary legislation or remedial order.

Proceedings.

7. - (1) A person who claims that a public authority has acted (or proposes to act) in a way which is made unlawful by section 6(1) may-

(a) bring proceedings against the authority under this Act in the appropriate court or tribunal, or
(b) rely on the Convention right or rights concerned in any legal proceedings,

but only if he is (or would be) a victim of the unlawful act.

(2) In subsection (1)(a) "appropriate court or tribunal" means such court or tribunal as may be determined in accordance with rules; and proceedings against an authority include a counterclaim or similar proceeding.

(3) If the proceedings are brought on an application for judicial review, the applicant is to be taken to have a sufficient interest in relation to the unlawful act only if he is, or would be, a victim of that act.

(4) If the proceedings are made by way of a petition for judicial review in Scotland, the applicant shall be

taken to have title and interest to sue in relation to the unlawful act only if he is, or would be, a victim of that act.

(5) Proceedings under subsection (1)(a) must be brought before the end of-

(a) the period of one year beginning with the date on which the act complained of took place; or
(b) such longer period as the court or tribunal considers equitable having regard to all the circumstances, but that is subject to any rule imposing a stricter time limit in relation to the procedure in question.

(6) In subsection (1)(b) "legal proceedings" includes-

(a) proceedings brought by or at the instigation of a public authority; and
(b) an appeal against the decision of a court or tribunal.

(7) For the purposes of this section, a person is a victim of an unlawful act only if he would be a victim for the purposes of Article 34 of the Convention if proceedings were brought in the European Court of Human Rights in respect of that act.

(8) Nothing in this Act creates a criminal offence.

(9) In this section "rules" means-

(a) in relation to proceedings before a court or tribunal outside Scotland, rules made by the Lord Chancellor or the Secretary of State for the purposes of this section or rules of court,
(b) in relation to proceedings before a court or tribunal in Scotland, rules made by the Secretary of State for those purposes,
(c) in relation to proceedings before a tribunal in Northern Ireland-
(i) which deals with transferred matters; and
(ii) for which no rules made under paragraph (a) are

in force, rules made by a Northern Ireland department for those purposes, and includes provision made by order under section 1 of the Courts and Legal Services Act 1990.

(10) In making rules, regard must be had to section 9.

(11) The Minister who has power to make rules in relation to a particular tribunal may, to the extent he considers it necessary to ensure that the tribunal can provide an appropriate remedy in relation to an act (or proposed act) of a public authority which is (or would be) unlawful as a result of section 6(1), by order add to-

(a) the relief or remedies which the tribunal may grant; or
(b) the grounds on which it may grant any of them.

(12) An order made under subsection (11) may contain such incidental, supplemental, consequential or transitional provision as the Minister making it considers appropriate.

(13) "The Minister" includes the Northern Ireland department concerned.

Judicial remedies.

8. - (1) In relation to any act (or proposed act) of a public authority which the court finds is (or would be) unlawful, it may grant such relief or remedy, or make such order, within its powers as it considers just and appropriate.

(2) But damages may be awarded only by a court which has power to award damages, or to order the payment of compensation, in civil proceedings.

(3) No award of damages is to be made unless, taking account of all the circumstances of the case,

including-

(a) any other relief or remedy granted, or order
    made, in relation to the act in question (by that or
    any other court), and
(b) the consequences of any decision (of that or any
    other court) in respect of that act,

the court is satisfied that the award is necessary to
afford just satisfaction to the person in whose
favour it is made.

(4) In determining-

(a) whether to award damages, or
(b) the amount of an award,

the court must take into account the principles
applied by the European Court of Human Rights in
relation to the award of compensation under Article
41 of the Convention.

(5) A public authority against which damages are
awarded is to be treated-

(a) in Scotland, for the purposes of section 3 of the
    Law Reform (Miscellaneous Provisions)
    (Scotland) Act 1940 as if the award were made in
    an action of damages in which the authority has
    been found liable in respect of loss or damage to
    the person to whom the award is made;
(b) for the purposes of the Civil Liability
    (Contribution) Act 1978 as liable in respect of
    damage suffered by the person to whom the
    award is made.

(6) In this section-

"court" includes a tribunal;
"damages" means damages for an unlawful act of a
public authority; and
"unlawful" means unlawful under section 6(1).

Judicial acts.

9. - (1) Proceedings under section 7(1)(a) in respect of a judicial act may be brought only-

(a) by exercising a right of appeal;
(b) on an application (in Scotland a petition) for judicial review; or
(c) in such other forum as may be prescribed by rules.

(2) That does not affect any rule of law which prevents a court from being the subject of judicial review.

(3) In proceedings under this Act in respect of a judicial act done in good faith, damages may not be awarded otherwise than to compensate a person to the extent required by Article 5(5) of the Convention.

(4) An award of damages permitted by subsection (3) is to be made against the Crown; but no award may be made unless the appropriate person, if not a party to the proceedings, is joined.

(5) In this section-

"appropriate person" means the Minister responsible for the court concerned, or a person or government department nominated by him;
"court" includes a tribunal;
"judge" includes a member of a tribunal, a justice of the peace and a clerk or other officer entitled to exercise the jurisdiction of a court;
"judicial act" means a judicial act of a court and includes an act done on the instructions, or on behalf, of a judge; and
"rules" has the same meaning as in section 7(9).

Remedial action
Power to take remedial action.

10. - (1) This section applies if-

(a) a provision of legislation has been declared
   under section 4 to be incompatible with a
   Convention right and, if an appeal lies-
(i) all persons who may appeal have stated in
   writing that they do not intend to do so;
(ii) the time for bringing an appeal has expired and
   no appeal has been brought within that time; or
(iii) an appeal brought within that time has been
   determined or abandoned; or
(b) it appears to a Minister of the Crown or Her
   Majesty in Council that, having regard to a finding
   of the European Court of Human Rights made
   after the coming into force of this section in
   proceedings against the United Kingdom, a
   provision of legislation is incompatible with an
   obligation of the United Kingdom arising from the
   Convention.

(2) If a Minister of the Crown considers that there
are compelling reasons for proceeding under this
section, he may by order make such amendments to
the legislation as he considers necessary to remove
the incompatibility.

(3) If, in the case of subordinate legislation, a Minister of the Crown considers-

(a) that it is necessary to amend the primary
   legislation under which the subordinate
   legislation in question was made, in order to
   enable the incompatibility to be removed, and
(b) that there are compelling reasons for proceeding
   under this section,

he may by order make such amendments to the
primary legislation as he considers necessary.

(4) This section also applies where the provision in
question is in subordinate legislation and has been
quashed, or declared invalid, by reason of incompatibility with a Convention right and the Minister proposes
to proceed under paragraph 2(b) of Schedule 2.

(5) If the legislation is an Order in Council, the power conferred by subsection (2) or (3) is exercisable by Her Majesty in Council.

(6) In this section "legislation" does not include a Measure of the Church Assembly or of the General Synod of the Church of England.

(7) Schedule 2 makes further provision about remedial orders.

Other rights and proceedings
Safeguard for existing human rights.

11. A person's reliance on a Convention right does not restrict-

(a) any other right or freedom conferred on him by or under any law having effect in any part of the United Kingdom; or
(b) his right to make any claim or bring any proceedings which he could make or bring apart from sections 7 to 9.

Freedom of expression.

12. - (1) This section applies if a court is considering whether to grant any relief which, if granted, might affect the exercise of the Convention right to freedom of expression.

(2) If the person against whom the application for relief is made ("the respondent") is neither present nor represented, no such relief is to be granted unless the court is satisfied-

(a) that the applicant has taken all practicable steps to notify the respondent; or
(b) that there are compelling reasons why the respondent should not be notified.

(3) No such relief is to be granted so as to restrain

publication before trial unless the court is satisfied that the applicant is likely to establish that publication should not be allowed.

(4) The court must have particular regard to the importance of the Convention right to freedom of expression and, where the proceedings relate to material which the respondent claims, or which appears to the court, to be journalistic, literary or artistic material (or to conduct connected with such material), to-

(a) the extent to which-
(i) the material has, or is about to, become available to the public; or
(ii) it is, or would be, in the public interest for the material to be published;
(b) any relevant privacy code.

(5) In this section-

"court" includes a tribunal; and
"relief" includes any remedy or order (other than in criminal proceedings).

Freedom of thought, conscience and religion.

13. - (1) If a court's determination of any question arising under this Act might affect the exercise by a religious organisation (itself or its members collectively) of the Convention right to freedom of thought, conscience and religion, it must have particular regard to the importance of that right.

(2) In this section "court" includes a tribunal.

Derogations and reservations
Derogations.

14. - (1) In this Act "designated derogation" means-

(a) the United Kingdom's derogation from Article 5(3) of the Convention; and

(b) any derogation by the United Kingdom from an Article of the Convention, or of any protocol to the Convention, which is designated for the purposes of this Act in an order made by the Secretary of State.

(2) The derogation referred to in subsection (1)(a) is set out in Part I of Schedule 3.

(3) If a designated derogation is amended or replaced it ceases to be a designated derogation.

(4) But subsection (3) does not prevent the Secretary of State from exercising his power under subsection (1)(b) to make a fresh designation order in respect of the Article concerned.

(5) The Secretary of State must by order make such amendments to Schedule 3 as he considers appropriate to reflect-

(a) any designation order; or
(b) the effect of subsection (3).

(6) A designation order may be made in anticipation of the making by the United Kingdom of a proposed derogation.

Reservations.

15. - (1) In this Act "designated reservation" means-

(a) the United Kingdom's reservation to Article 2 of the First Protocol to the Convention; and
(b) any other reservation by the United Kingdom to an Article of the Convention, or of any protocol to the Convention, which is designated for the purposes of this Act in an order made by the Secretary of State.

(2) The text of the reservation referred to in subsection (1)(a) is set out in Part II of Schedule 3.

(3) If a designated reservation is withdrawn wholly or in part it ceases to be a designated reservation.

(4) But subsection (3) does not prevent the Secretary of State from exercising his power under subsection (1)(b) to make a fresh designation order in respect of the Article concerned.

(5) The Secretary of State must by order make such amendments to this Act as he considers appropriate to reflect-

(a) any designation order; or
(b) the effect of subsection (3).

Period for which designated derogations have effect.

16. - (1) If it has not already been withdrawn by the United Kingdom, a designated derogation ceases to have effect for the purposes of this Act-

(a) in the case of the derogation referred to in section 14(1)(a), at the end of the period of five years beginning with the date on which section 1(2) came into force;
(b) in the case of any other derogation, at the end of the period of five years beginning with the date on which the order designating it was made.

(2) At any time before the period-

(a) fixed by subsection (1)(a) or (b), or
(b) extended by an order under this subsection,

comes to an end, the Secretary of State may by order extend it by a further period of five years.

(3) An order under section 14(1)(b) ceases to have effect at the end of the period for consideration, unless a resolution has been passed by each House approving the order.

(4) Subsection (3) does not affect-

(a) anything done in reliance on the order; or
(b) the power to make a fresh order under section
    14(1)(b).

(5) In subsection (3) "period for consideration"
means the period of forty days beginning with the
day on which the order was made.

(6) In calculating the period for consideration, no
account is to be taken of any time during which-

(a) Parliament is dissolved or prorogued; or
(b) both Houses are adjourned for more than four
    days.

(7) If a designated derogation is withdrawn by the
United Kingdom, the Secretary of State must by
order make such amendments to this Act as he
considers are required to reflect that withdrawal.

Periodic review of designated reservations.

17. - (1) The appropriate Minister must review the
designated reservation referred to in section
15(1)(a)-

(a) before the end of the period of five years
    beginning with the date on which section 1(2)
    came into force; and
(b) if that designation is still in force, before the end
    of the period of five years beginning with the date
    on which the last report relating to it was laid
    under subsection (3).

(2) The appropriate Minister must review each of the
other designated reservations (if any)-

(a) before the end of the period of five years
    beginning with the date on which the order

designating the reservation first came into force; and

(b) if the designation is still in force, before the end of the period of five years beginning with the date on which the last report relating to it was laid under subsection (3).

(3) The Minister conducting a review under this section must prepare a report on the result of the review and lay a copy of it before each House of Parliament.

Judges of the European Court of Human Rights

Appointment to European Court of Human Rights.

18. - (1) In this section "judicial office" means the office of-

(a) Lord Justice of Appeal, Justice of the High Court or Circuit judge, in England and Wales;
(b) judge of the Court of Session or sheriff, in Scotland;
(c) Lord Justice of Appeal, judge of the High Court or county court judge, in Northern Ireland.

(2) The holder of a judicial office may become a judge of the European Court of Human Rights ("the Court") without being required to relinquish his office.

(3) But he is not required to perform the duties of his judicial office while he is a judge of the Court.

(4) In respect of any period during which he is a judge of the Court-

(a) a Lord Justice of Appeal or Justice of the High Court is not to count as a judge of the relevant court for the purposes of section 2(1) or 4(1) of the Supreme Court Act 1981 (maximum number of judges) nor as a judge of the Supreme Court for the purposes of section 12(1) to (6) of that Act (salaries etc.);

(b) a judge of the Court of Session is not to count as a judge of that court for the purposes of section 1(1) of the Court of Session Act 1988 (maximum number of judges) or of section 9(1)(c) of the Administration of Justice Act 1973 ("the 1973 Act") (salaries etc.);

(c) a Lord Justice of Appeal or judge of the High Court in Northern Ireland is not to count as a judge of the relevant court for the purposes of section 2(1) or 3(1) of the Judicature (Northern Ireland) Act 1978 (maximum number of judges) nor as a judge of the Supreme Court of Northern Ireland for the purposes of section 9(1)(d) of the 1973 Act (salaries etc.);

(d) a Circuit judge is not to count as such for the purposes of section 18 of the Courts Act 1971 (salaries etc.);

(e) a sheriff is not to count as such for the purposes of section 14 of the Sheriff Courts (Scotland) Act 1907 (salaries etc.);

(f) a county court judge of Northern Ireland is not to count as such for the purposes of section 106 of the County Courts Act Northern Ireland) 1959 (salaries etc.).

(5) If a sheriff principal is appointed a judge of the Court, section 11(1) of the Sheriff Courts (Scotland) Act 1971 (temporary appointment of sheriff principal) applies, while he holds that appointment, as if his office is vacant.

(6) Schedule 4 makes provision about judicial pensions in relation to the holder of a judicial office who serves as a judge of the Court.

(7) The Lord Chancellor or the Secretary of State may by order make such transitional provision (including, in particular, provision for a temporary increase in the maximum number of judges) as he considers appropriate in relation to any holder of a judicial office who has completed his service as a judge of the Court.

Parliamentary procedure
Statements of compatibility.

> **19.** - (1) A Minister of the Crown in charge of a Bill in either House of Parliament must, before Second Reading of the Bill-
>
> (a) make a statement to the effect that in his view the provisions of the Bill are compatible with the Convention rights ("a statement of compatibility"); or
> (b) make a statement to the effect that although he is unable to make a statement of compatibility the government nevertheless wishes the House to proceed with the Bill.
>
> (2) The statement must be in writing and be published in such manner as the Minister making it considers appropriate.

Supplemental
Orders etc. under this Act.

> **20.** - (1) Any power of a Minister of the Crown to make an order under this Act is exercisable by statutory instrument.
>
> (2) The power of the Lord Chancellor or the Secretary of State to make rules (other than rules of court) under section 2(3) or 7(9) is exercisable by statutory instrument.
>
> (3) Any statutory instrument made under section 14, 15 or 16(7) must be laid before Parliament.
>
> (4) No order may be made by the Lord Chancellor or the Secretary of State under section 1(4), 7(11) or 16(2) unless a draft of the order has been laid before, and approved by, each House of Parliament.
>
> (5) Any statutory instrument made under section 18(7) or Schedule 4, or to which subsection (2)

applies, shall be subject to annulment in pursuance of a resolution of either House of Parliament.

(6) The power of a Northern Ireland department to make-

(a) rules under section 2(3)(c) or 7(9)(c), or
(b) an order under section 7(11),

is exercisable by statutory rule for the purposes of the Statutory Rules (Northern Ireland) Order 1979.

(7) Any rules made under section 2(3)(c) or 7(9)(c) shall be subject to negative resolution; and section 41(6) of the Interpretation Act (Northern Ireland) 1954 (meaning of "subject to negative resolution") shall apply as if the power to make the rules were conferred by an Act of the Northern Ireland Assembly.

(8) No order may be made by a Northern Ireland department under section 7(11) unless a draft of the order has been laid before, and approved by, the Northern Ireland Assembly.

Interpretation, etc.

21. - (1) In this Act-

"amend" includes repeal and apply (with or without modifications);
"the appropriate Minister" means the Minister of the Crown having charge of the appropriate authorised government department (within the meaning of the Crown Proceedings Act 1947);
"the Commission" means the European Commission of Human Rights;
"the Convention" means the Convention for the Protection of Human Rights and Fundamental Freedoms, agreed by the Council of Europe at Rome on 4th November 1950 as it has effect for the time being in relation to the United Kingdom;

"declaration of incompatibility" means a declaration under section 4;

"Minister of the Crown" has the same meaning as in the Ministers of the Crown Act 1975;

"Northern Ireland Minister" includes the First Minister and the deputy First Minister in Northern Ireland;

"primary legislation" means any-

(a) public general Act;

(b) local and personal Act;

(c) private Act;

(d) Measure of the Church Assembly;

(e) Measure of the General Synod of the Church of England;

(f) Order in Council-

(i) made in exercise of Her Majesty's Royal Prerogative;

(ii) made under section 38(1)(a) of the Northern Ireland Constitution Act 1973 or the corresponding provision of the Northern Ireland Act 1998; or

(iii) amending an Act of a kind mentioned in paragraph (a), (b) or (c);

and includes an order or other instrument made under primary legislation (otherwise than by the National Assembly for Wales, a member of the Scottish Executive, a Northern Ireland Minister or a Northern Ireland department) to the extent to which it operates to bring one or more provisions of that legislation into force or amends any primary legislation;

"the First Protocol" means the protocol to the Convention agreed at Paris on 20th March 1952;

"the Sixth Protocol" means the protocol to the Convention agreed at Strasbourg on 28th April 1983;

"the Eleventh Protocol" means the protocol to the Convention (restructuring the control machinery established by the Convention) agreed at Strasbourg on 11th May 1994;

"remedial order" means an order under section 10;

"subordinate legislation" means any-

(a) Order in Council other than one-
(i) made in exercise of Her Majesty's Royal
    Prerogative;
(ii) made under section 38(1)(a) of the Northern
     Ireland Constitution Act 1973 or the
     corresponding provision of the Northern Ireland
     Act 1998; or
(iii)amending an Act of a kind mentioned in the
     definition of primary legislation;
(b) Act of the Scottish Parliament;
(c) Act of the Parliament of Northern Ireland;
(d) Measure of the Assembly established under
    section 1 of the Northern Ireland Assembly Act
    1973;
(e) Act of the Northern Ireland Assembly;
(f) order, rules, regulations, scheme, warrant,
    byelaw or other instrument made under primary
    legislation (except to the extent to which it
    operates to bring one or more provisions of that
    legislation into force or amends any primary
    legislation);
(g) order, rules, regulations, scheme, warrant,
    byelaw or other instrument made under
    legislation mentioned in paragraph (b), (c), (d) or
    (e) or made under an Order in Council applying
    only to Northern Ireland;
(h) order, rules, regulations, scheme, warrant,
    byelaw or other instrument made by a member of
    the Scottish Executive, a Northern Ireland
    Minister or a Northern Ireland department in
    exercise of prerogative or other executive
    functions of Her Majesty which are exercisable by
    such a person on behalf of Her Majesty;
"transferred matters" has the same meaning as in
the Northern Ireland Act 1998; and
"tribunal" means any tribunal in which legal proceedings may be brought.

(2) The references in paragraphs (b) and (c) of
section 2(1) to Articles are to Articles of the Convention as they had effect immediately before the
coming into force of the Eleventh Protocol.

(3) The reference in paragraph (d) of section 2(1) to Article 46 includes a reference to Articles 32 and 54 of the Convention as they had effect immediately before the coming into force of the Eleventh Protocol.

(4) The references in section 2(1) to a report or decision of the Commission or a decision of the Committee of Ministers include references to a report or decision made as provided by paragraphs 3, 4 and 6 of Article 5 of the Eleventh Protocol (transitional provisions).

(5) Any liability under the Army Act 1955, the Air Force Act 1955 or the Naval Discipline Act 1957 to suffer death for an offence is replaced by a liability to imprisonment for life or any less punishment authorised by those Acts; and those Acts shall accordingly have effect with the necessary modifications.

Short title, commencement, application and extent.

22. - (1) This Act may be cited as the Human Rights Act 1998.

(2) Sections 18, 20 and 21(5) and this section come into force on the passing of this Act.

(3) The other provisions of this Act come into force on such day as the Secretary of State may by order appoint; and different days may be appointed for different purposes.

(4) Paragraph (b) of subsection (1) of section 7 applies to proceedings brought by or at the instigation of a public authority whenever the act in question took place; but otherwise that subsection does not apply to an act taking place before the coming into force of that section.

(5) This Act binds the Crown.

(6) This Act extends to Northern Ireland.

(7) Section 21(5), so far as it relates to any provision contained in the Army Act 1955, the Air Force Act 1955 or the Naval Discipline Act 1957, extends to any place to which that provision extends.

Schedule 1

THE ARTICLES
PART I
THE CONVENTION

RIGHTS AND FREEDOMS

ARTICLE 2   *RIGHT TO LIFE*
1. Everyone's right to life shall be protected by law. No one shall be deprived of his life intentionally save in the execution of a sentence of a court following his conviction of a crime for which this penalty is provided by law.

2. Deprivation of life shall not be regarded as inflicted in contravention of this Article when it results from the use of force which is no more than absolutely necessary:

(a) in defence of any person from unlawful violence;
(b) in order to effect a lawful arrest or to prevent the escape of a person lawfully detained;
(c) in action lawfully taken for the purpose of quelling a riot or insurrection.

ARTICLE 3   *PROHIBITION OF TORTURE*
No one shall be subjected to torture or to inhuman or degrading treatment or punishment.

ARTICLE 4   *PROHIBITION OF SLAVERY AND FORCED LABOUR*
1. No one shall be held in slavery or servitude.

2. No one shall be required to perform forced or compulsory labour.

3. For the purpose of this Article the term "forced or compulsory labour" shall not include:

(a) any work required to be done in the ordinary course of detention imposed according to the provisions of Article 5 of this Convention or during conditional release from such detention;
(b) any service of a military character or, in case of conscientious objectors in countries where they are recognised, service exacted instead of compulsory military service;
(c) any service exacted in case of an emergency or calamity threatening the life or well-being of the community;
(d) any work or service which forms part of normal civic obligations.

ARTICLE 5   *RIGHT TO LIBERTY AND SECURITY*
1. Everyone has the right to liberty and security of person. No one shall be deprived of his liberty save in the following cases and in accordance with a procedure prescribed by law:

(a) the lawful detention of a person after conviction by a competent court;
(b) the lawful arrest or detention of a person for non-compliance with the lawful order of a court or in order to secure the fulfilment of any obligation prescribed by law;
(c) the lawful arrest or detention of a person effected for the purpose of bringing him before the competent legal authority on reasonable suspicion of having committed an offence or when it is reasonably considered necessary to prevent his committing an offence or fleeing after having done so;
(d) the detention of a minor by lawful order for the purpose of educational supervision or his lawful detention for the purpose of bringing him before the competent legal authority;
(e) the lawful detention of persons for the prevention of the spreading of infectious diseases, of

persons of unsound mind, alcoholics or drug
addicts or vagrants;

(f) the lawful arrest or detention of a person to prevent
his effecting an unauthorised entry into the country
or of a person against whom action is being taken
with a view to deportation or extradition.

2. Everyone who is arrested shall be informed
promptly, in a language which he understands, of
the reasons for his arrest and of any charge against
him.

3. Everyone arrested or detained in accordance with
the provisions of paragraph 1(c) of this Article shall
be brought promptly before a judge or other officer
authorised by law to exercise judicial power and
shall be entitled to trial within a reasonable time or
to release pending trial. Release may be conditioned
by guarantees to appear for trial.

4. Everyone who is deprived of his liberty by arrest
or detention shall be entitled to take proceedings by
which the lawfulness of his detention shall be
decided speedily by a court and his release ordered
if the detention is not lawful.

5. Everyone who has been the victim of arrest or
detention in contravention of the provisions of this Article shall have an enforceable right to compensation.

ARTICLE 6   *RIGHT TO A FAIR TRIAL*
1. In the determination of his civil rights and obligations or of any criminal charge against him, everyone is entitled to a fair and public hearing within a
reasonable time by an independent and impartial
tribunal established by law. Judgment shall be
pronounced publicly but the press and public may be
excluded from all or part of the trial in the interest of
morals, public order or national security in a democratic society, where the interests of juveniles or the
protection of the private life of the parties so

require, or to the extent strictly necessary in the opinion of the court in special circumstances where publicity would prejudice the interests of justice.

2. Everyone charged with a criminal offence shall be presumed innocent until proved guilty according to law.

3. Everyone charged with a criminal offence has the following minimum rights:

(a) to be informed promptly, in a language which he understands and in detail, of the nature and cause of the accusation against him;
(b) to have adequate time and facilities for the preparation of his defence;
(c) to defend himself in person or through legal assistance of his own choosing or, if he has not sufficient means to pay for legal assistance, to be given it free when the interests of justice so require;
(d) to examine or have examined witnesses against him and to obtain the attendance and examination of witnesses on his behalf under the same conditions as witnesses against him;
(e) to have the free assistance of an interpreter if he cannot understand or speak the language used in court.

ARTICLE 7   *NO PUNISHMENT WITHOUT LAW*
1. No one shall be held guilty of any criminal offence on account of any act or omission which did not constitute a criminal offence under national or international law at the time when it was committed. Nor shall a heavier penalty be imposed than the one that was applicable at the time the criminal offence was committed.

2. This Article shall not prejudice the trial and punishment of any person for any act or omission which, at the time when it was committed, was criminal according to the general principles of law recognised by civilised nations.

ARTICLE 8   *RIGHT TO RESPECT FOR PRIVATE AND FAMILY LIFE*
1. Everyone has the right to respect for his private and family life, his home and his correspondence.

2. There shall be no interference by a public authority with the exercise of this right except such as is in accordance with the law and is necessary in a democratic society in the interests of national security, public safety or the economic well-being of the country, for the prevention of disorder or crime, for the protection of health or morals, or for the protection of the rights and freedoms of others.

ARTICLE 9   *FREEDOM OF THOUGHT, CONSCIENCE AND RELIGION*
1. Everyone has the right to freedom of thought, conscience and religion; this right includes freedom to change his religion or belief and freedom, either alone or in community with others and in public or private, to manifest his religion or belief, in worship, teaching, practice and observance.

2. Freedom to manifest one's religion or beliefs shall be subject only to such limitations as are prescribed by law and are necessary in a democratic society in the interests of public safety, for the protection of public order, health or morals, or for the protection of the rights and freedoms of others.

ARTICLE 10   *FREEDOM OF EXPRESSION*
1. Everyone has the right to freedom of expression. This right shall include freedom to hold opinions and to receive and impart information and ideas without interference by public authority and regardless of frontiers. This Article shall not prevent States from requiring the licensing of broadcasting, television or cinema enterprises.

2. The exercise of these freedoms, since it carries with it duties and responsibilities, may be subject to such formalities, conditions, restrictions or penalties as are prescribed by law and are necessary in a

democratic society, in the interests of national security, territorial integrity or public safety, for the prevention of disorder or crime, for the protection of health or morals, for the protection of the reputation or rights of others, for preventing the disclosure of information received in confidence, or for maintaining the authority and impartiality of the judiciary.

ARTICLE 11   *FREEDOM OF ASSEMBLY AND ASSOCIATION*
1. Everyone has the right to freedom of peaceful assembly and to freedom of association with others, including the right to form and to join trade unions for the protection of his interests.

2. No restrictions shall be placed on the exercise of these rights other than such as are prescribed by law and are necessary in a democratic society in the interests of national security or public safety, for the prevention of disorder or crime, for the protection of health or morals or for the protection of the rights and freedoms of others. This Article shall not prevent the imposition of lawful restrictions on the exercise of these rights by members of the armed forces, of the police or of the administration of the State.

ARTICLE 12   *RIGHT TO MARRY*
Men and women of marriageable age have the right to marry and to found a family, according to the national laws governing the exercise of this right.

ARTICLE 14   *PROHIBITION OF DISCRIMINATION*
The enjoyment of the rights and freedoms set forth in this Convention shall be secured without discrimination on any ground such as sex, race, colour, language, religion, political or other opinion, national or social origin, association with a national minority, property, birth or other status.

ARTICLE 16   *RESTRICTIONS ON POLITICAL ACTIVITY OF ALIENS*
Nothing in Articles 10, 11 and 14 shall be regarded as preventing the High Contracting Parties from

imposing restrictions on the political activity of aliens.

ARTICLE 17   *PROHIBITION OF ABUSE OF RIGHTS*
Nothing in this Convention may be interpreted as implying for any State, group or person any right to engage in any activity or perform any act aimed at the destruction of any of the rights and freedoms set forth herein or at their limitation to a greater extent than is provided for in the Convention.

ARTICLE 18   *LIMITATION ON USE OF RESTRICTIONS ON RIGHTS*
The restrictions permitted under this Convention to the said rights and freedoms shall not be applied for any purpose other than those for which they have been prescribed.

PART II
THE FIRST PROTOCOL
ARTICLE 1   *PROTECTION OF PROPERTY*
Every natural or legal person is entitled to the peaceful enjoyment of his possessions. No one shall be deprived of his possessions except in the public interest and subject to the conditions provided for by law and by the general principles of international law.
The preceding provisions shall not, however, in any way impair the right of a State to enforce such laws as it deems necessary to control the use of property in accordance with the general interest or to secure the payment of taxes or other contributions or penalties.

ARTICLE 2   *RIGHT TO EDUCATION*
No person shall be denied the right to education. In the exercise of any functions which it assumes in relation to education and to teaching, the State shall respect the right of parents to ensure such education and teaching in conformity with their own religious and philosophical convictions.

ARTICLE 3   *RIGHT TO FREE ELECTIONS*
The High Contracting Parties undertake to hold free elections at reasonable intervals by secret ballot, under conditions which will ensure the free expression of the opinion of the people in the choice of the legislature.

PART III
THE SIXTH PROTOCOL

ARTICLE 1   *ABOLITION OF THE DEATH PENALTY*
The death penalty shall be abolished. No one shall be condemned to such penalty or executed.

ARTICLE 2   *DEATH PENALTY IN TIME OF WAR*
A State may make provision in its law for the death penalty in respect of acts committed in time of war or of imminent threat of war; such penalty shall be applied only in the instances laid down in the law and in accordance with its provisions. The State shall communicate to the Secretary General of the Council of Europe the relevant provisions of that law.

Schedule 2
REMEDIAL ORDERS

Orders

1. - (1) A remedial order may-

(a) contain such incidental, supplemental, consequential or transitional provision as the person making it considers appropriate;
(b) be made so as to have effect from a date earlier than that on which it is made;
(c) make provision for the delegation of specific functions;
(d) make different provision for different cases.

(2) The power conferred by sub-paragraph (1)(a) includes-

(a) power to amend primary legislation (including primary legislation other than that which contains

the incompatible provision); and

(b) power to amend or revoke subordinate legislation (including subordinate legislation other than that which contains the incompatible provision).

(3) A remedial order may be made so as to have the same extent as the legislation which it affects.

(4) No person is to be guilty of an offence solely as a result of the retrospective effect of a remedial order.

Procedure

2. No remedial order may be made unless-

(a) a draft of the order has been approved by a resolution of each House of Parliament made after the end of the period of 60 days beginning with the day on which the draft was laid; or

(b) it is declared in the order that it appears to the person making it that, because of the urgency of the matter, it is necessary to make the order without a draft being so approved.

Orders laid in draft

3. - (1) No draft may be laid under paragraph 2(a) unless-

(a) the person proposing to make the order has laid before Parliament a document which contains a draft of the proposed order and the required information; and

(b) the period of 60 days, beginning with the day on which the document required by this sub-paragraph was laid, has ended.

(2) If representations have been made during that period, the draft laid under paragraph 2(a) must be accompanied by a statement containing-

(a) a summary of the representations; and

(b) if, as a result of the representations, the

proposed order has been changed, details of the changes.

Urgent cases

4. - (1) If a remedial order ("the original order") is made without being approved in draft, the person making it must lay it before Parliament, accompanied by the required information, after it is made.

(2) If representations have been made during the period of 60 days beginning with the day on which the original order was made, the person making it must (after the end of that period) lay before Parliament a statement containing-

(a) a summary of the representations; and
(b) if, as a result of the representations, he considers it appropriate to make changes to the original order, details of the changes.

(3) If sub-paragraph (2)(b) applies, the person making the statement must-

(a) make a further remedial order replacing the original order; and
(b) lay the replacement order before Parliament.

(4) If, at the end of the period of 120 days beginning with the day on which the original order was made, a resolution has not been passed by each House approving the original or replacement order, the order ceases to have effect (but without that affecting anything previously done under either order or the power to make a fresh remedial order).

Definitions

5. In this Schedule-

"representations" means representations about a remedial order (or proposed remedial order) made to the person making (or proposing to make) it and includes any relevant Parliamentary report or resolution; and

"required information" means-
(a) an explanation of the incompatibility which the
    order (or proposed order) seeks to remove,
    including particulars of the relevant declaration,
    finding or order; and
(b) a statement of the reasons for proceeding under
    section 10 and for making an order in those
    terms.

Calculating periods

6. In calculating any period for the purposes of this
Schedule, no account is to be taken of any time
during which-

(a) Parliament is dissolved or prorogued; or
(b) both Houses are adjourned for more than four
    days.

Schedule 3
DEROGATION AND RESERVATION

PART I
DEROGATION

The 1988 notification

The United Kingdom Permanent Representative to
the Council of Europe presents his compliments to
the Secretary General of the Council, and has the
honour to convey the following information in order
to ensure compliance with the obligations of Her
Majesty's Government in the United Kingdom under
Article 15(3) of the Convention for the Protection of
Human Rights and Fundamental Freedoms signed at
Rome on 4 November 1950.

There have been in the United Kingdom in recent
years campaigns of organised terrorism connected
with the affairs of Northern Ireland which have mani-
fested themselves in activities which have included
repeated murder, attempted murder, maiming, intim-
idation and violent civil disturbance and in bombing
and fire raising which have resulted in death, injury

and widespread destruction of property. As a result, a public emergency within the meaning of Article 15(1) of the Convention exists in the United Kingdom.

The Government found it necessary in 1974 to introduce and since then, in cases concerning persons reasonably suspected of involvement in terrorism connected with the affairs of Northern Ireland, or of certain offences under the legislation, who have been detained for 48 hours, to exercise powers enabling further detention without charge, for periods of up to five days, on the authority of the Secretary of State. These powers are at present to be found in Section 12 of the Prevention of Terrorism (Temporary Provisions) Act 1984, Article 9 of the Prevention of Terrorism (Supplemental Temporary Provisions) Order 1984 and Article 10 of the Prevention of Terrorism (Supplemental Temporary Provisions) (Northern Ireland) Order 1984.

Section 12 of the Prevention of Terrorism (Temporary Provisions) Act 1984 provides for a person whom a constable has arrested on reasonable grounds of suspecting him to be guilty of an offence under Section 1, 9 or 10 of the Act, or to be or to have been involved in terrorism connected with the affairs of Northern Ireland, to be detained in right of the arrest for up to 48 hours and thereafter, where the Secretary of State extends the detention period, for up to a further five days. Section 12 substantially re-enacted Section 12 of the Prevention of Terrorism (Temporary Provisions) Act 1976 which, in turn, substantially re-enacted Section 7 of the Prevention of Terrorism (Temporary Provisions) Act 1974.

Article 10 of the Prevention of Terrorism (Supplemental Temporary Provisions) (Northern Ireland) Order 1984 (SI 1984/417) and Article 9 of the Prevention of Terrorism (Supplemental Temporary Provisions) Order 1984 (SI 1984/418) were both made under Sections 13 and 14 of and Schedule 3 to the 1984 Act and substantially re-enacted powers of detention in Orders made under the 1974 and 1976 Acts. A person who is being examined under

Article 4 of either Order on his arrival in, or on seeking to leave, Northern Ireland or Great Britain for the purpose of determining whether he is or has been involved in terrorism connected with the affairs of Northern Ireland, or whether there are grounds for suspecting that he has committed an offence under Section 9 of the 1984 Act, may be detained under Article 9 or 10, as appropriate, pending the conclusion of his examination. The period of this examination may exceed 12 hours if an examining officer has reasonable grounds for suspecting him to be or to have been involved in acts of terrorism connected with the affairs of Northern Ireland.

Where such a person is detained under the said Article 9 or 10 he may be detained for up to 48 hours on the authority of an examining officer and thereafter, where the Secretary of State extends the detention period, for up to a further five days.

In its judgment of 29 November 1988 in the Case of *Brogan and Others*, the European Court of Human Rights held that there had been a violation of Article 5(3) in respect of each of the applicants, all of whom had been detained under Section 12 of the 1984 Act. The Court held that even the shortest of the four periods of detention concerned, namely four days and six hours, fell outside the constraints as to time permitted by the first part of Article 5(3). In addition, the Court held that there had been a violation of Article 5(5) in the case of each applicant.

Following this judgment, the Secretary of State for the Home Department informed Parliament on 6 December 1988 that, against the background of the terrorist campaign, and the over-riding need to bring terrorists to justice, the Government did not believe that the maximum period of detention should be reduced. He informed Parliament that the Government were examining the matter with a view to responding to the judgment. On 22 December 1988, the Secretary of State further informed Parliament that it remained the Government's wish, if it could be achieved, to find a judicial process under which extended detention might be reviewed and where appropriate authorised by a judge or other judicial officer. But a further period of reflection and consultation was necessary before the Government could bring forward a firm and final view.

Since the judgment of 29 November 1988 as well as previously, the Government have found it necessary to continue to exercise, in relation to terrorism connected with the affairs of Northern Ireland, the powers described above enabling further detention without charge for periods of up to 5 days, on the authority of the Secretary of State, to the extent strictly required by the exigencies of the situation to enable necessary enquiries and investigations properly to be completed in order to decide whether criminal proceedings should be instituted. To the extent that the exercise of these powers may be inconsistent with the obligations imposed by the Convention the Government has availed itself of the right of derogation conferred by Article 15(1) of the Convention and will continue to do so until further notice.

Dated 23 December 1988.

The 1989 notification

The United Kingdom Permanent Representative to the Council of Europe presents his compliments to the Secretary General of the Council, and has the honour to convey the following information.

In his communication to the Secretary General of 23 December 1988, reference was made to the introduction and exercise of certain powers under section 12 of the Prevention of Terrorism (Temporary Provisions) Act 1984, Article 9 of the Prevention of Terrorism (Supplemental Temporary Provisions) Order 1984 and Article 10 of the Prevention of Terrorism (Supplemental Temporary Provisions) (Northern Ireland) Order 1984.

These provisions have been replaced by section 14 of and paragraph 6 of Schedule 5 to the Prevention of Terrorism (Temporary Provisions) Act 1989, which make comparable provision. They came into force on 22 March 1989. A copy of these provisions is enclosed.

The United Kingdom Permanent Representative avails himself of this opportunity to renew to the Secretary General the assurance of his highest consideration.

23 March 1989.

PART II
RESERVATION

At the time of signing the present (First) Protocol, I declare that, in view of certain provisions of the Education Acts in the United Kingdom, the principle affirmed in the second sentence of Article 2 is accepted by the United Kingdom only so far as it is compatible with the provision of efficient instruction and training, and the avoidance of unreasonable public expenditure.

Dated 20 March 1952

Made by the United Kingdom Permanent Representative to the Council of Europe.

Schedule 4
JUDICIAL PENSIONS

Duty to make orders about pensions

1. - (1) The appropriate Minister must by order make provision with respect to pensions payable to or in respect of any holder of a judicial office who serves as an ECHR judge.

(2) A pensions order must include such provision as the Minister making it considers is necessary to secure that-

(a) an ECHR judge who was, immediately before his appointment as an ECHR judge, a member of a judicial pension scheme is entitled to remain as a member of that scheme;

(b) the terms on which he remains a member of the scheme are those which would have been applicable had he not been appointed as an ECHR judge; and

(c) entitlement to benefits payable in accordance with the scheme continues to be determined as if, while serving as an ECHR judge, his salary was that which would (but for section 18(4)) have been payable to him in respect of his continuing service as the holder of his judicial office.

Contributions

2. A pensions order may, in particular, make provision-

(a) for any contributions which are payable by a person who remains a member of a scheme as a result of the order, and which would otherwise be payable by deduction from his salary, to be made otherwise than by deduction from his salary as an ECHR judge; and

(b) for such contributions to be collected in such manner as may be determined by the administrators of the scheme.

Amendments of other enactments

3. A pensions order may amend any provision of, or made under, a pensions Act in such manner and to such extent as the Minister making the order considers necessary or expedient to ensure the proper administration of any scheme to which it relates.

Definitions

4. In this Schedule-

"appropriate Minister" means-

(a) in relation to any judicial office whose jurisdiction is exercisable exclusively in relation to Scotland, the Secretary of State; and

(b) otherwise, the Lord Chancellor;

"ECHR judge" means the holder of a judicial office who is serving as a judge of the Court;
"judicial pension scheme" means a scheme established by and in accordance with a pensions Act;

"pensions Act" means-
(a) the County Courts Act (Northern Ireland) 1959;
(b) the Sheriffs' Pensions (Scotland) Act 1961;
(c) the Judicial Pensions Act 1981; or
(d) the Judicial Pensions and Retirement Act 1993;

and "pensions order" means an order made under paragraph 1.

Appendix 2: Summary of the Convention rights incorporated into the Human Rights Act 1998

Article	Right	Absolute/ qualified
2	Right to life	A
3	Right not to be subjected to torture or inhuman treatment	A
4	Right to freedom from slavery or forced labour	A
5	Right to liberty and security of person	Q
6	Right to a fair trial	A
7	Right to non-respective criminal laws	A
8	Right to respect for private and family life, home and correspondence	Q
9	Right to freedom of thought, conscience and religion	Q
10	Right to freedom of expression	Q
11	Right to freedom of peaceful assembly and freedom of association	Q
12	Right to marry and found a family	A
14	Right not to be discriminated against in the enjoyment of the rights and freedoms in the Act	Q
16	Exception to rights in Articles 10,11 and 14 in relation to restricting the political activities of aliens	Q
17	Prohibition of abuse of Convention rights	Q
18	Limitation on use of restrictions on rights permitted by the Convention	Q
The First Protocol, Article 1	Right to peaceful enjoyment of possessions	Q
The First Protocol, Article 2	Right to education	Q
The First Protocol, Article 3	Right to free elections	A
The Sixth Protocol Articles 1 and 2	Abolition of the death penalty except in times of war or imminent threat of war	A

Appendix 3: ICN's Code of Ethics for Nurses

An international code of ethics for nurses was first adopted by the International Council of Nurses (ICN) in 1953. It has been revised and reaffirmed at various times since, most recently with this review and revision, which was completed in 2000. It is printed here with permission from ICN. http://www.icn.ch

Preamble

Nurses have four fundamental responsibilities: to promote health, to prevent illness, to restore health and to alleviate suffering. The need for nursing is universal.

Inherent in nursing is respect for human rights, including the right to life, to dignity and to be treated with respect.

Nursing care is unrestricted by considerations of age, colour, creed, culture, disability or illness, gender, nationality, politics, race or social status.

Nurses render health services to the individual, the family and the community and co-ordinate their services with those of related groups.

THE CODE

The ICN Code of Ethics for Nurses has four principal elements that outline the standards of ethical conduct.

1. Nurses and people

The nurse's primary professional responsibility is to people requiring nursing care.

In providing care, the nurse promotes an environment in which the human rights, values, customs and spiritual beliefs of the individual, family and community are respected.

The nurse ensures that the individual receives sufficient information on which to base consent for care and related treatment.

The nurse holds in confidence personal information and uses judgement in sharing this information.

The nurse shares with society the responsibility for initiating and supporting action to meet the health and social needs of the public, in particular those of vulnerable populations.

The nurse also shares responsibility to sustain and protect the natural environment from depletion, pollution, degradation and destruction.

2. Nurses and practice

The nurse carries personal responsibility and accountability for nursing practice, and for maintaining competence by continual learning.

The nurse maintains a standard of personal health such that the ability to provide care is not compromised.

The nurse uses judgement regarding individual competence when accepting and delegating responsibility.

The nurse at all times maintains standards of personal conduct which reflect well on the profession and enhance public confidence.

The nurse, in providing care, ensures that use of technology and scientific advances are compatible with the safety, dignity and rights of people.

3. Nurses and the profession

The nurse assumes the major role in determining and implementing acceptable standards of clinical nursing practice, management, research and education.

The nurse is active in developing a core of research-based professional knowledge.

The nurse, acting through the professional organisation, participates in creating and maintaining equitable social and economic working conditions in nursing.

4. Nurses and co-workers

The nurse sustains a co-operative relationship with co-workers in nursing and other fields.

The nurse takes appropriate action to safeguard individuals when their care is endangered by a co-worker or any other person.

Suggestions for use of the *ICN Code of Ethics for Nurses*

The *ICN Code of Ethics for Nurses* is a guide for action based on social values and needs. It will have meaning only as a living document if applied to the realities of nursing and health care in a changing society.

To achieve its purpose the Code must be understood, internalised and used by nurses in all aspects of their work. It must be available to students and nurses throughout their study and work lives.

The full ICN Code contains further suggestions and charts for applying the Elements of the Code. Details can be found on the ICN website: www.icn.ch/mal

References

ANA (1991) Ethics and Human Rights. Position statement. American Nurses
    Association. www.nursingworld.org/ethics/index.html
Being Heard: The Report of a Review Committee on NHS Complaints Procedures (1994)
    DO16/BH/10M. London: Department of Health.
Chester M (1998) Human Rights in the Health Service. Association of Community
    Health Councils for England and Wales.
Chester M (2000) Human Rights Issues. Association of Community Health Councils for
    England and Wales.
CNA (1991) Human Rights. Position statement on human rights. Canadian Nurses
    Association. www.cna-nurses.ca/pages/policies/human_rights.hml
European Social Charter 1998 Recommendation 1354 (1998) Future of the European
    Social Charter.
Herman L, Fuenzalida-Puelma HL, Scholle S (1989) The Right to Health in the
    Americas, Scientific Publication No. 509. Washington DC: Pan-American Health
    Organization.
ICN (1998) Nurses and Human Rights. ICN position statement. Geneva: International
    Council of Nurses.
ICN (1999) ICN on Health and Human Rights, ICN/99/8. Geneva: International
    Council of Nurses.
Iliffe S, Munro J (1997) Healthy Choices: Future Options for the NHS. London:
    Lawrence & Wishart.
Lord Irvine (1998) The patient, the doctor, their lawyers and the judge: rights and duties.
    The Long Fox lecture. November, Bristol University.
NHS Executive (1996) Complaints, Listening ... Acting ... Improving: Guidance on
    Implementation of the NHS Complaints Procedure. London HMSO.
NHS (1977) National Health Service Act 1977 cited in Ferraz OLM (2000) Health care
    as a human right. Dispatches, 9(3): 12–13.
NHS (2000) The NHS Plan: A Plan for Investment, A Plan for Reform. London:
    HMSO.
Reidy A (1999) The Human Rights ImpAct on Health Care. Seminar Discussion Paper
    given at Nuffield Trust, London, November.
Rights Brought Home: the Human Rights Bill (1997) London: HMSO.
Rivett G (1997) From Cradle to Grave: Fifty Years of the NHS. London: Kings Fund.
Straw J (2000) Human Rights Act. Speech given at IPPR Conference, Impact of the
    Human Rights Act on the private and voluntary sectors, March, London.

UKCC (1992) Code of Professional Conduct. London: United Kingdom Central Council.

UNISON (2000) Human Rights: UNISON's Guide to the Human Rights Act 1998, www.unison.org.uk

WHO (1998) Health for all: towards the 21st century. Agenda Item 19 at 51st World Health Assembly, May.

WHO (2000) World Health Report 2000, www.who.rnt/whr/2000/en/report.htm

Index

IN FOCUS

ANTHROPOLOGY AND HUMAN RIGHTS

"[C]ompeting and divergent perspectives on anthropology and human rights make this one of the areas of anthropology that is ripe for renewed attention, especially in light of the underlying stakes involved," wrote Mark Goodale, assistant professor of conflict analysis and anthropology at George Mason University, in his introduction to the AN series on Anthropology and Human Rights he guest edits. In this AN series spanning from April until October 2006, people from a range of different backgrounds and perspectives respond to one of four questions: Do anthropologists have anything useful or relevant to say about human rights? (April)

Should anthropologists try and answer whether human rights are universal? (May) Is the spread of human rights discourse since the end of the Cold War a form of moral imperialism? (Sept) And, do anthropologists have an ethical obligation to promote human rights? (Oct)

Is the Spread of Human Rights Discourse Since the End of the Cold War a Form of Moral Imperialism?

Human Rights and Moral Imperialism

A Double-Edged Story

LAURA NADER
UC BERKELEY

ncreasingly anthropologists are writing about human rights from a critical perspective, documenting how human rights organizations may operate as facilitators

gies and cultures. Yet in the commission there were no representatives from the indigenous peoples of the world, from the so-called Third World, from the peoples of Islam, and little input from women in spite of Roosevelt's presence.

With all due respect for her one world, Roosevelt belonged to an era of women reformers, women who viewed their positions as possible role models for other capable, educated women. They were social

Rights of Women

Normative blindness is never more obvious than in Western dealings with the rights of women, elsewhere. For example, the actions and accusations of human rights activists waiting to liberate Islamic women was used as a justification for preemptive war during the Gulf conflict, then the invasion of Afghanistan, then Iraq—to liberate

Comparison Needed

Not long ago a headline in the New York Times noted that 25% of Syrian men beat their wives. At a World Bank conference I noted people reporting that Bolivian men beat their wives. Could this be related to axis-of-evil politics? Comparative figures would reveal that American domestic violence is about the same as Syria—25%.

requires that we look at ourselves as well as those others whose plight moves us to reach out while ironically also ensuring that we are blinded.

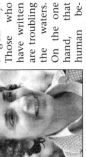

Laura Nader

Those who have written are troubling the waters. On the one hand, that human be-ings have rights to air, water and life because they are human seems obvious. On the other, interventions by human rights activists or truth commissions can and do have hurtful consequences. In other words, there is a double edge to the human rights story.

Normative Blindness

The exercise of power through the categorization of knowledge requires an understanding of how the human rights movement started. The human rights movement had its beginnings at the end of WWII. As chairperson of the UN Human Rights Commission, Eleanor Roosevelt insisted that the declarations had to be acceptable to peoples of all religions, ideolo-tion, the movement to create a new international apparatus for human rights promotion was led largely by Americans. The US State Department orchestrated the early drafts and the crucial meetings took place in the US.

The generalities were unassailable: Everyone has a right to life, liberty and security of person; freedom of thought, conscience and religion; no one shall be held in slavery, subjected to torture, subjected to arbitrary arrest, detention or exile. And all but two drafts were written in English. It was definitely a paradigm open to interpretation, especially with the presupposition that international human rights standards are culturally neutral. For these reasons the human rights lens is bound to find violations of human rights that point to deficiencies elsewhere.

From the beginning human rights are something Euro-Americans take to others. Richard Falk, a scholar who has distinguished himself for his lucidity on human rights issues, labels the problem one of normative blindness—a blindness that accompanies a modernization outlook, one that regards premodern cultures as a form of backwardness that needs to be overcome.

Islamic women. Islam and Islamic women are essentialized.

Afghan women are presumably like Iraqi women—both repressed and in need of help from more modern countries. Even ethnographic work has not articulated effectively the differences from place to place—for example, Iraqi women under Saddam Hussein were the most equal in the professions like medicine, law and engineering than any other Arab country, and there were more women in engineering classes in Baghdad University that at UC Berkeley during the same time period. Basically anthropological writings have been case by case—now Saudi Arabia, now Iran, now Morocco, analyzing status regimes. But our work did not compare Islamic realities with American realities.

Perhaps they should appear in the same article along with the observation that assaults by husbands, ex-husbands and lovers cause more injuries to women than motor vehicle accidents, rape and muggings combined.

It's about time that anthropologists used such comparisons to support the public health observation that male-dominated society is a threat to public health *everywhere*. The credibility of a human rights spirit requires that we look at ourselves as well as those others whose plight moves us to reach out while ironically also ensuring that we are blinded. ∎

Laura Nader's current work focuses on how central dogmas are made and how they work in law, energy science and anthropology.